INTRODUCING
IMMUNOLOGY

INTRODUCING
IMMUNOLOGY
SECOND EDITION

Norman A Staines BSc, PhD
Professor of Immunology
Immunology and Parasitology Group
King's College London
Campden Hill Road, London W8 7AH

Jonathan Brostoff MA, DM(Oxon), DSc, FRCP, FRCPath
Reader in Clinical Immunology
Department of Immunology
University College London Medical School
Arthur Stanley House
40–50 Tottenham Street, London W9 9PG

Keith James PhD, DSc, FRCPath, FRSE
Professor of Immunology
Department of Surgery
The Medical School, University of Edinburgh
Teviot Place, Edinburgh EH8 9AG

M Mosby
St. Louis Baltimore Boston Chicago London Philadelphia Sydney Toronto

Project Manager	Michael Smith
Design and Illustration	Timothy Read
Linework	Marion Tasker, Lee Smith
Production	Jane Tozer
Index	Nina Boyd
Publisher	Fiona Foley

A *Slide Atlas of Introducing Immunology,* based on the contents of this book, is available. In the slide atlas format, the material is presented in a binder, together with numbered 35mm slides of each illustration. Further information is available from the publishers.

For full details of Mosby-Yearbook Europe Limited titles please write to:
Mosby-Yearbook Europe Limited
Lynton House
7–12 Tavistock Square
London WC1H 9LB
England

Cataloguing-in-Publications Data:
Cataloguing records for this book are available from the US Library of Congress and the British Library.

ISBN: 0 397 44734 5

Typeset in New Baskerville, legends set in Gill Sans
Produced by China Translation and Printing Services Limited
Printed and bound in Hong Kong, 1993

Cover illustration: A scanning electron micrograph of an HIV-infected T-helper cell ($\times$20,000). Courtesy of D Hockley.

PREFACE

Immunology is a science of great public importance. It enjoys wide exposure in the media and enormous attention from the scientific community. We all know about immunity to infection, but it goes beyond that. It is hard, perhaps impossible, to think of a disease, or group of diseases, that does not in some way involve an aspect of immunology. This tells you how important the immune system is to your health.

The language of immunology, like that of all special subjects, is difficult and our purpose in writing this book is to explain it. In doing this, we hope to stimulate you with the subject that has devoured our attention for all our working scientific lives, and will no doubt continue to do so.

This is the second edition of the book. The first was published in 1985, with the encouragement and support of the British Society for Immunology, with the idea of making immunology accessible to students in schools, colleges and universities. It was the warm response that the first book received that has encouraged us to write this version now in your hands.

Much has changed, but this book is still harnessed firmly to its title – it is to introduce immunology to you. There are many excellent books that will take you further, but this is to get you started. Progress in our subject has been so rapid that we cannot do justice to it without covering a wide area. So, the book is bigger than before and is now more illustrated. One of the reasons for this is that we will make a slide set of the illustrations that will help our many colleagues who have told us how much they valued the first edition of *Introducing Immunology* in teaching the subject.

The jargon of science is kept under as much control as we can manage, and there is a glossary of terms to refer to. We explain new words when they first appear in the text. The figures and their captions are self-contained but they also support the text. Where we go into detail that was missing in the first edition we do so because much more is now understood and the topics are important.

As authors it is a pleasure to acknowledge the generous advice of our friends and colleagues in the scientific, medical and teaching communities and the help, support and professionalism of many at Gower Medical Publishing, but especially Fiona Foley who nursed the project and encouraged the authors, Michael Smith who managed the project and Tim Read for the design and illustration.

Immunology grows and evolves at a pace that catches even immunologists unawares. This is for many the excitement of the subject. In our first edition we included a section at the end that we called Frontiers of Immunology. Looking back at this, everything discussed there has become well established and is now incorporated in the text of this edition. That alone tells us it was time to write this new book for you. Here, we include throughout the text many of the exciting things happening today in experimental immunology that we believe will soon be exploited in clinical practice.

We say welcome to our regular readers and send a special greeting to new ones: this is for you and we hope you enjoy it.

Norman Staines
Jonathan Brostoff
Keith James   1993

CONTENTS

IMMUNE RESPONSES

CONTENTS

INTRODUCTION

Are you one of those lucky individuals who rarely seem to catch the colds and other common infections which repeatedly plague your friends? If this is so, it is because you have a very efficient immune system. This is an intricate system of cells which functions in a variety of ways to make you resistant or immune to infection by microorganisms and other large parasites. This resistance may be acquired as a result of chance exposure to infectious agents or as a consequence of deliberate immunization.

The reactions of the immune system to infectious agents are crucial to survival and hence they are usually beneficial for your continued health. They either prevent infection or ensure that infections are limited or eradicated without causing long-lasting or deleterious effects. Sometimes, however, there is a price to pay for this vital protection, with the control of infection being at the expense of some damage (usually transient) to the tissues in which the microorganisms are located. Furthermore, in some people the immune system may malfunction giving rise to unpleasant over reactions which can seriously damage rather than protect the body. These include common conditions such as hay fever, allergies to foods, cosmetics and drugs, and a plethora of diseases collectively known as autoimmune diseases in which the immune system attacks the body's own tissues. A common example of the latter is rheumatoid arthritis in which over-reactivity of the immune system leads to damage of the joints.

Underactivity of the immune system may be equally serious because it can lead to an increased susceptibility to infection. In a few people it is due to inherent defects in the immune system itself, while in others it may be a direct consequence of the use of drugs which suppress the immune system, such as those routinely used to prevent graft rejection in transplant patients. Malnutrition also leads to decreased immunity as is so frequently seen in the Third World. Deficiencies of particular nutrients, for example zinc, also lead to diminished immune responses. Finally, it has become very clear recently that some viruses may seriously impair the cells of the immune system, thus predisposing the body to infection. The best known is the human immunodeficiency virus (HIV) which gives rise to AIDS, the acquired immunodeficiency syndrome.

The science of immunology is the study of the immune system; how it works, how it reacts, what happens when it goes wrong and how it can be manipulated for our benefit. As a result of the outstanding efforts of scientists from a wide range of backgrounds, immunology has made great advances in recent years and will undoubtedly continue to do so. Biochemists and chemists, molecular biologists and geneticists, zoologists and veterinarians, physicians and surgeons, have all played their part.

Nobel Prizes and Immunology		
Year	Nobel Laureate	Discovery or invention
1901	Emil von Behring	Serum immunotherapy
1905	Robert Koch	Discovery of tubercle bacillus and tuberculin
1908	Paul Ehrlich Elie Metchnikoff	Mechanisms of phagocytosis Theories of antibody formation
1913	Charles Richet	Discovery of anaphylaxis
1919	Jules Bordet	Mechanisms of complement-mediated haemolysis
1930	Karl Landsteiner	Discovery of human blood groups
1951	Max Theiler	Vaccines against yellow fever
1957	Daniel Bovet	Antihistamines for treatment of allergy
1960	F. MacFarlane Burnet & Peter B. Medawar	Acquired immunological tolerance
1972	Rodney R. Porter & Gerald M. Edelman	Chemical structure of antibodies
1977	Rosalyn Yalow	Development of radioimmunoassays for peptide hormones
1980	Baruj Benaceraff, Jean Dausset & George Snell	Function of the major histocompatability complex
1984	Cesar Milstein & Georges F. Köhler	How to make monoclonal antibodies
	Niels K. Jerne	Theories of immune system function
1987	Susumu Tonegawa	Genetic basis of antibody diversity
1990	Joseph Murray	Contributions to kidney transplantation
	Donell Thomas	Successful transplantation of human bone marrow

2

The relevance of immunology to humanity is highlighted by the fact that on 15 occasions this century the Nobel Prize has been awarded to individuals who have advanced its understanding and practice (Table 1). In recent years this honour has been bestowed upon investigators who have increased our knowledge of the mechanisms of transplant rejection, the structure of antibody molecules and the genetic control of the immune response. Others have developed novel techniques for producing immunological reagents of immense value in the diagnosis and treatment of disease. Most recently it was awarded to Joseph Murray and Donnell Thomas for their outstanding contributions to human kidney and bone marrow transplantation, respectively.

While the rapid advance of our subject clearly owes much to the endeavours of those trained in other disciplines, it has given much to them in return. Apart from the immunological techniques that are widely used in many areas of science and medicine, the immune system itself has provided a rich source of material for investigating basic aspects of cell and molecular biology. It has, for example, provided model systems for studying the development, activation and intricate interactions of cells and the complex control of protein synthesis.

There is still, however, much to be learned about the immune system and still more remains to be exploited for the benefit of mankind. We need a fuller understanding of immune reactions at the molecular and cellular level and this will continue to require the concerted efforts of scientists of different disciplines. An even greater challenge lies in developing ways to selectively manipulate various parts of the immune response. This requires the dedicated effort of clinical and non-clinical scientists alike and could be of inestimable value in the prevention and treatment of many diseases.

In this book we aim to introduce this important and obviously complex subject to a wide audience. It will acquaint you with the basic organization and working of the immune system. We also highlight the central importance of the immune system to health, what happens when it goes wrong and how it can be manipulated for the benefit of mankind. Finally, we want to persuade you to develop your interest in this subject and to realize that a career in immunology can be both exciting and rewarding.

IMMUNITY AND COMPONENTS OF THE IMMUNE SYSTEM

The immune system is a collection of tissues, cells and molecules whose prime physiological function is to maintain the internal environment of the body by destroying invading infectious organisms. However, the immune system also has other important related functions that are not concerned with fighting infection. For example, cells of the immune system contribute to wound healing and aid the removal of cells that die through natural processes.

The Dynamic Interaction of the Immune System

The immune system does not operate in isolation. This is one of its cardinal features. It interacts with all the other physiological systems such as the neuroendocrine, gastrointestinal, respiratory, urogenital, and musculoskeletal systems. The cells of the immune system are distributed throughout every part of the body, and indeed, many of them actively travel or 'migrate' around it.

In order to understand the immune system it is important to realize that it interacts in a dynamic way with all the tissues of the body. As a consequence of these interactions, the proper functioning of the immune system is essential to the proper functioning of the body as a whole. When the immune system malfunctions, other parts of the body may suffer, and in turn, disturbances elsewhere may perturb the immune system and influence our resistance to infection. For example, people who have Cushing's syndrome produce abnormally high amounts of adrenal corticosteroid hormone (cortisone) which suppresses the activity of their immune system. As a result, these patients suffer more than usual from infections. Understanding these intricate relationships is one of the great challenges of immunology.

The skin and the linings of the respiratory, gastrointestinal and urogenital tracts present formidable physical and chemical barriers to infective organisms and represent a first line of defence. These barriers provide a natural immunity, sometimes called *innate immunity*, to infection but they are, however, less than perfect. Microorganisms have evolved in such a way that they resist destruction or physical removal and penetrate the body's defences, particularly at the site of an injury. It is after this that the cells of the immune system come into play. They recognize the microorganisms and mount an immune response against them which neutralizes or destroys them. As a result, the immune system itself becomes altered: the next time it is exposed to the same microorganism it reacts more quickly and aggressively than the first time. This is known as a *secondary immune response* and indicates a state of *acquired immunity* to infection. This acquired (or adaptive) immunity also has the peculiar property of being specific for the microorganism in question. In these respects it is quite unlike natural immunity which is nonspecific and does not change with repeated exposure to the same microorganism. Thus, acquired immunity is characterized by specific immunological *memory* (Table 2).

Contrasting properties of natural and acquired immunity		
	Natural	Acquired
Resistance	Unaltered on repeated infection	Improved by repeated infection (= memory)
Specificity	Generally effective against all organisms	Specific for stimulating organism
Important cells	Phagocytes Natural killer cells	Lymphocytes
Important molecules	Lysozyme Complement Acute phase proteins Interferons	Antibodies Cytokines from lymphocytes

Table 2. Contrasting properties of natural and acquired immunity. Although we conveniently classify immunity into these two broad arms, it is essential to remember that the agents of natural and acquired immunity interact intimately with each other. Natural immunity is the more primitive evolutionarily, and you can think of the mechanisms of acquired immunity all being directed to amplifying and making more efficient the mechanisms of natural immunity. Remember the central importance of phagocytosis in protective immunity of all types.

Natural and Adaptive Immune Functions

It is largely a matter of convenience that we think of these as separate forms of immunity. In reality the mechanisms of natural and acquired immunity are inextricably connected with each other. The mechanisms of natural immunity provide the basic means for the destruction of infectious microorganisms (to simplify matters we will use this term to refer to all classes of infectious agents), and the mechanisms of acquired immunity provide powerful ways to improve and enhance the efficiency of natural mechanisms and to remember the infection the next time it is encountered.

We are all familiar with the value of *vaccination*: it produces a state of acquired immunity and it nicely illustrates what is meant by the term specific. Vaccination, for example with poliomyelitis virus, induces resistance to later infection by poliomyelitis virus but not to infection by influenza virus. This sort of immunity is specific and highly discriminatory for different microorganisms. The development of a universal vaccine against the common cold is proving to be very difficult because so many different strains of the virus cause colds without individually inducing any useful immunity against each other. We will discuss this later when we deal with immunity to virus infections.

Protection Against Infection

In understanding how the immune system protects us against infectious disease it is as well to realize that there is a dynamic relationship between our body – the host – and the infectious microorganism – the invader. The evolutionary pressures exerted by infection have meant that the immune system has evolved into the form that we can now see in mammals, that has many different ways of dealing with microorganisms. In turn, some organisms have responded to the skill and sophistication of the immune system and its responses by developing tricks to avoid being attacked by immune mechanisms. We will discuss many of these later on, but an important and topical example is HIV that is associated with AIDS. In common with all viruses, HIV spends most of its life hidden inside cells, in this case cells of the immune system, so that it is not 'seen' by the immune system. Although immune responses are made against the proteins of the virus, they do not directly interact with the hidden virus and so they really are not very effective at eliminating it. The malarial parasite, probably responsible for more deaths annually than any other parasite, hides inside red blood cells and liver cells so that it also cannot be attacked easily by the immune system. While malarial organisms are exposed to attack

7

during their life cycle when they are outside cells, they change
the proteins of their surface at this time which makes it hard for
the immune system to recognize and react to them quickly
enough before they go back inside other cells.

Antigens

Materials which induce specific immune reactions are called
antigens; most are not normal constituents of our bodies. In addition to the antigen molecules of microorganisms and parasites
there appears to be no limit to the range of materials that can
behave as antigens. Proteins, carbohydrates, lipids, nucleic acids,
organic compounds and inorganic compounds can all induce
immune reactions. At first sight this may appear startling, but it
is probably the inevitable consequence of the evolutionary development of an adaptive immune system capable of reacting to an
equally startling and large range of microorganisms.

Lymphocytes

The specialized cells of the immune system which recognize antigens are called *lymphocytes.* After recognizing an antigen, lymphocytes can react in a variety of ways. Some lymphocytes secrete
proteins called *antibodies* into the blood and body fluids.
Antibodies combine with the antigen that the lymphocytes
reacted to initially, leading eventually to the destruction or
removal of the antigen. Other lymphocytes do not secrete antibodies, but instead directly destroy cells or parasites bearing the
antigens to which they react. Yet other lymphocytes produce substances which in turn activate other cells, some of which in their
turn regulate the activity of the lymphocytes which reacted to the
initial antigen!

Self and Non-Self

In describing the role of the immune system there has always
been the notion that it is very effective at reacting to foreign
antigens but not to self antigens. In other words it is capable of
discriminating between our own body, 'self', and foreign
materials, 'non-self'. This idea has its roots in the earliest days of
the science of immunology, and it is undoubtedly correct in the
sense that the normally functioning immune system reacts aggressively against foreign antigens but not against self, even though
self molecules may be very similar in structure to the foreign molecules. However, one of the exciting realizations of recent
research has been the demonstration that even totally healthy
individuals do possess lymphocytes that have the potential to
react to self antigens. The fact that they do not actually do so very

often tells us that these cells are under some special form of control that prevents this happening. When they do respond they are said to make autoallergic or autoimmune reactions, and these can sometimes cause *autoimmune disease*. As mentioned earlier, the immune system has important roles in wound healing and clearing cell debris and therefore the ability to react to self can, under certain circumstances, be a useful homeostatic attribute.

Careful study of the development of the immune system has shown that many of the lymphocytes present in embryos and in newborn humans and animals are autoreactive. It seems that this type of reactivity is well developed before the individual becomes capable of reacting to foreign antigens. However, not all auto-reactive cells survive for very long, and it is clear that the *thymus* has an important role in this. It is the graveyard in which most developing lymphocytes die, many of which are thought to be autoreactive. This deletion of unwanted cells ensures that most of the dangerous cells do not persist to cause disease. We shall return to this later.

Historically, antibodies were the first components of the immune system, as we understand it today, to be found to have a role in acquired immunity. Only later was it realized that lympho-cytes produced antibodies and that these lymphocytes circulate throughout the body and are organized into lymphoid tissues. These collectively make up the lymphoid system. The thymus is one of the primary lymphoid tissues (the bone marrow is the other) and it must have been known long ago – the Greeks of classical times thought it to be the seat of the soul – but its immune function has only been appreciated within the last forty years. We will now consider some of the important molecules and cells that participate in natural and acquired immunity, and will later explain how these are organized and how they function.

NATURAL IMMUNITY

EXTERNAL SURFACES

The horny layer of the skin and the membranous linings of the various body tracts provide formidable physical and chemical bar-riers to infectious agents (Figure 1). Acids are widely secreted by these linings and enzymes such as *lysozyme*, which digests bacterial cell walls, are found in mucus and tears. Mucus is composed mainly of mucins, long branched carbohydrate molecules that are rather acidic, and it is the combination of these physical proper-ties that makes them especially good at sticking to and trapping invading microorganisms. This can prevent the organisms from

9

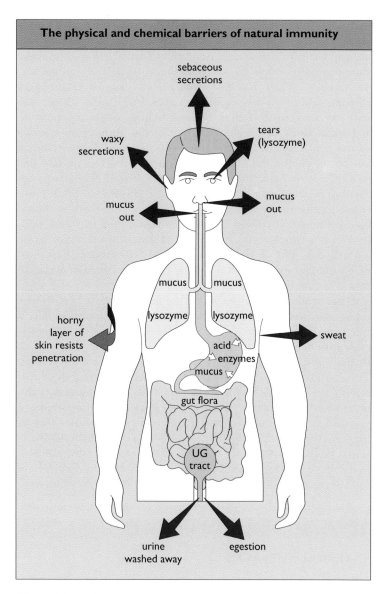

Figure 1. The physical and chemical barriers of natural immunity.
The skin provides a formidable physical barrier to microorganisms and its
secretions are also microbicidal. The mucosal surfaces, whose normal
physiological functions are absorptive, require the special protection provided
by the secretion of mucus and enzymes like lysozyme. If any of these external
surfaces are breached, then a variety of cells and secreted molecules provides
rapid protection against infection. The effectiveness of these natural
mechanisms of immunity does not change with repeated exposure to infection.

attaching to receptors on lining epithelial cells by which they would normally invade the tissues, and it may lead to their physical expulsion in the mucus that, for example, can be washed out of the lungs by the beating of cilia on epithelial cells in the respiratory tract (Figure 2a). Coughing and sneezing are also highly effective ways of expelling foreign materials trapped in mucus; they are also highly effective ways of spreading infection! The importance of so-called *mucous membranes* in preventing infection can be appreciated by studying the disease cystic fibrosis. Here, a viscous form of mucus is produced which is not protective and this leads to chronic persistent respiratory infections which may eventually be fatal.

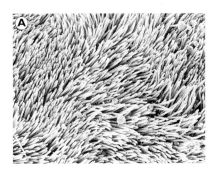

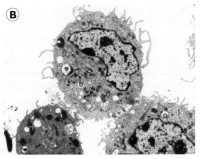

Figure 2. The ciliated cells of the respiratory tract.
(A) Ciliated cells lining the respiratory tract. The beating of the cilia move the mucus containing particles and microorganisms trapped within it up the trachea. Damage to these cells prevents the expulsion of these undesirable invaders. Scanning electron micrograph courtesy of Andrew Rutman. (B) The alveoli of the lungs themselves contain many phagocytic cells in the air spaces. Their job is to ingest foreign particles as can be seen in the inclusions in the alveolar cells illustrated. Particles may later be pumped out of the lungs with the mucus. Electron micrograph courtesy of Wangxue Chen, MR Alley and BW Manktelow.

Healthy humans have many symbiotic bacteria resident in their gastrointestinal and urinogenitary tracts. They do not cause disease but interestingly they may prevent pathogenic microorganisms from growing because they compete, with overwhelming success, for nutrients. This process is known as microbial antagonism and it can be severely disturbed in some people who take antibiotics orally. If these drugs kill the resident symbiotic bacteria, severe infections can arise such as thrush, which is caused by the fungus *Candida albicans*.

INTERNAL TISSUES

If organisms do penetrate the body then there are a number of anti-microbial agents that can be produced or activated rapidly in response to infection. These are all non-specific in their effects in that they are equally effective against many different groups of microorganisms, for example, bacteria or viruses. These agents include lysozyme, *acute phase proteins* and the *interferons*. The acute phase proteins are a diverse group of proteins, many of which are made by cells of the liver, examples are C-reactive protein, serum amyloid, orosomucoid and lactoferrin. Some have complex structures and many have combining sites for binding to various foreign materials. This may allow them to promote the phagocytosis of foreign material. Although in some cases their real importance is not understood, it is clear that they are synthesized rapidly in the liver in response to *inflammation* at distant sites. This introduces you to inflammation as one of the central features of protective immune responses to infection.

The interferons (IFNs) are probably better understood than the acute phase proteins. They are members of a large and diverse family, discovered originally through their ability to inhibit the replication of viruses inside cells. Some (IFN-α and IFN-β) may be synthesized by a cell as a direct consequence of its infection with virus, showing that their function is to prevent the spread of infection and to limit infection of the same cell with more than one type of virus (superinfection). However, some interferons (IFN-β and IFN-γ) are produced by lymphocytes in response to their stimulation by antigen and they have functions that extend beyond being anti-viral. Thus, they are not only agents of natural immunity but are also involved in mediating acquired immunity. The importance of interferons may be understood when it is remembered that, while replicating inside cells, viruses themselves are hidden from lymphocytes.

PHAGOCYTIC CELLS

The ultimate fate of foreign materials entering the body is probably ingestion and destruction by phagocytic cells (Figure 3). Two groups of cells phagocytose microorganisms. The first are the *polymorphonuclear neutrophil leucocytes* (PMNs), known as polymorphs or neutrophils. They circulate in the blood and migrate into the tissues very quickly in response to a local invasion by microorganisms. The second are the *monocytes* of the blood and the *macrophages* which reside in all body tissues and which are collectively referred to as the monocyte-macrophage system (previously the reticulo-endothelial system) (Figure 4). The liver, *spleen*, lungs (Figure 2b), kidney and *lymph nodes* have large

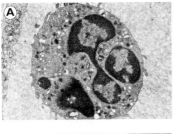
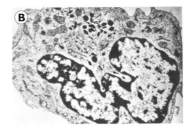
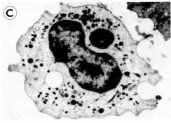

Figure 3. The phagocytic cells.
Electron micrographs of (A) a neutrophil, (B) a blood monocyte and (C) a macrophage.

numbers of macrophages and these are all tissues through which blood and lymph pass. Thus they provide sites of filtration where microorganisms can be removed from the circulation.

Cell Migration

One of the impressive features of the immune system is the mobility of its cells. As we shall see, lymphocytes originate in the bone marrow and migrate to different tissues, largely through the blood. A critical step in the migration of cells such as PMNs and monocytes from the blood to the tissues is their adherence to the vascular endothelial cells that line the walls of blood vessels. Cells generally adhere to each other because they possess particular molecules on their surface, referred to collectively as *adhesion molecules*, that interact with each other. There are many examples of these and they are involved whenever cells of the immune system interact with each other and with the cells of other tissues.

After adhesion to the endothelium, the phagocytic cells then migrate between the endothelial cells, cross through the basement membrane of the blood vessel and enter the tissues. This is the so-called process of diapedesis and is illustrated in Figure 5. The critical importance of adhesion molecules in this process is revealed by the rare defect known as leucocyte adhesion deficiency in which one adhesion molecule, known as CD18, is not expressed on the cell surface. In children severely affected with

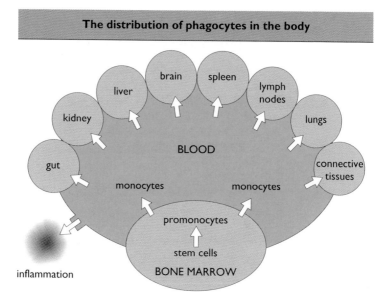

Figure 4. The distribution of phagocytes in the body.
All cells of the monocyte-macrophage system arise from stem cells in the bone marrow. These cells divide under the influence of colony-stimulating factors (see Table 3) that stimulate myelopoiesis. Promonocytes leave the bone marrow and travel through the blood as monocytes to settle in all tissues of the body, where they are collectively referred to as macrophages. Those in the spleen, liver and kidney remove material from the blood stream, those in the lymph nodes deal with materials brought in by the afferent lymph. The others serve local specialized functions to deal with invasive microorganisms. Circulating monocytes leave the blood by traversing the vascular endothelium, and their accumulation in sites of inflammation may be provoked by chemotactic factors that include complement components. Note that polymorphs (not illustrated) are also derived from the same multipotent stem cells. However, unlike macrophages, PMNs survive for relatively short periods and are produced and enter the tissues in response to acute inflammatory stimuli.

this disorder, PMNs and other leucocytes do not leave the blood to enter the tissues in response to local infection and as a result they suffer from recurrent life-threatening bacterial infections.

Phagocytosis and Killing
The mechanism of phagocytosis (or endocytosis) is well known to biologists. Macrophages eat bacteria in just the same way that amoebae eat food particles. They recognize foreign material, bind it to their cell membrane and engulf it in a membrane-lined vacuole. Ingested bacteria are killed within these vacuoles,

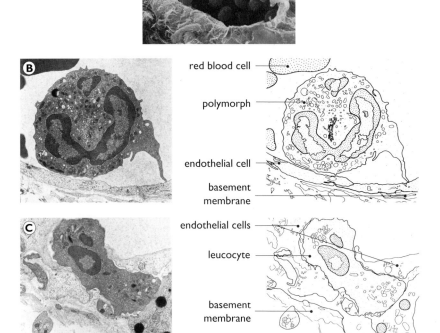

red blood cell

polymorph

endothelial cell

basement membrane

endothelial cells

leucocyte

basement membrane

Figure 5. The migration of leucocytes through blood vessel walls.
There are four stages in this process. First, leucocytes roll along the surface of the endothelial cells that line the vessel (A). This leads to the second stage in which both cells become activated and express new molecules on their surfaces. This enables the leucocytes to adhere to the endothelial cells. This is the third stage, illustrated here by the transmission electron micrograph of a leucocyte adhering to the wall of a vessel passing through inflamed tissue (B). The final stage involves the leucocytes squeezing between the endothelial cells and passing through the basement membrane to enter the tissues in response to chemotactic stimuli (C).

probably through the generation of toxic inorganic radicals and then digested by lysosomal enzymes (Figure 6).

Not only can phagocytes destroy material after it has been ingested but they can also kill other cells and some parasites without phagocytosis by a process of extracellular killing. We will look later at these mechanisms of *cytotoxicity*, but it is interesting in the context of natural immunity to point out that a particular

15

population of *large granular lymphocytes* (LGL) also has this property of killing other cells (Figure 7). These are known as *natural killer (NK) cells* and they are probably important in destroying some virus-infected cells. They also are thought to destroy cells of some types of tumours and in this way they have a role in the *immune surveillance* of tissue cells for malignant changes. Finally, they have what is considered a non-immunological function in

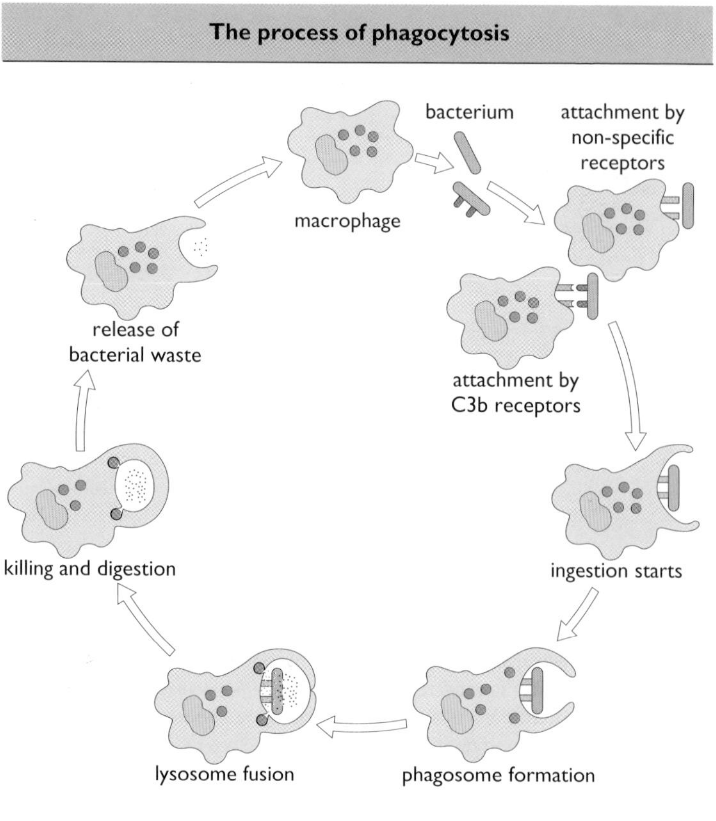

The process of phagocytosis

Figure 6. The process of phagocytosis.
The stages illustrated show how the foreign particle, here a bacterium, first adheres to the cell membrane of the macrophage. Various receptors facilitate this process, including receptors for complement components (or antibodies) that have coated the bacterium. As a response to binding the bacterium to its receptors, the cell membrane invaginates to form a pocket (receptor-mediated endocytosis) that isolates the particle inside a vesicle (phagosome) inside the cell. This fuses with lysosomes and the production of toxic chemicals and release of oxygen kill and digest the bacterium. The cell egests the remnants and is all the time available to eat other particles.

controlling the growth and proliferation of *stem cells* in bone marrow that give rise to some of the circulating cells in the blood. The efficiency with which microorganisms are phagocytosed is increased by antibodies and components of the *complement system* which bind first to the surface of the organism. The complement system, as described later, is a highly complex molecular cascade. Components of it initiate inflammation, increase permeability of tissues to blood plasma proteins and can directly kill invading microorganisms

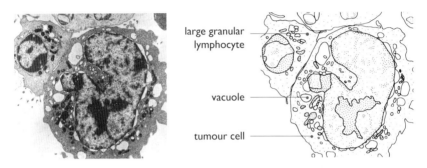

large granular lymphocyte

vacuole

tumour cell

Figure 7. Extracellular killing by a large granular lymphocyte.
Here, a large granular lymphocyte attaches to the cell membrane of a larger tumour cell. Through a complicated process, it damages the membrane of the tumour cell which makes it leaky – bubbles of fluid enter it making vacuoles as the first stage of the fatal process that destroys it. Killing similar to this, although differing in its detailed mechanism, is also used by macrophages, eosinophils and T-cytotoxic cells as a way of destroying various types of parasites or virus-infected cells.

ACQUIRED IMMUNITY

We have stressed the fundamental importance of the mechanisms of natural immunity, and we will now consider the ways in which immune cells contribute to acquired immunity. The features of acquired immunity, which distinguish it from natural immunity, are that immune responses are specific for individual stimulating antigens, that many diverse specific responses can be made and that the process of making a response leads to an altered state of immunity – referred to as memory – that ensures a subsequent response to the same stimulus is more powerful and more quickly made. Therefore, *specificity*, diversity and memory are the key features of acquired immunity (see Table 2). To explain how such responses are generated we will first deal with the nature of the cells and tissues of the immune system. **17**

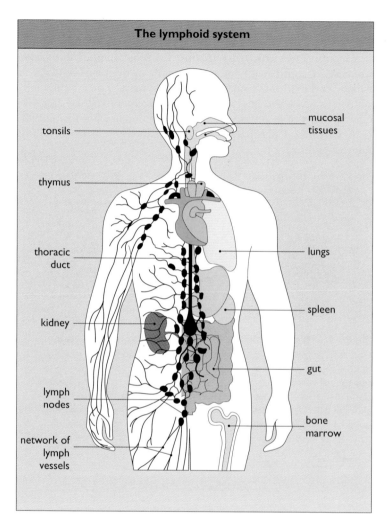

The lymphoid system

tonsils

thymus

thoracic
duct

kidney

lymph
nodes

network of
lymph
vessels

mucosal
tissues

lungs

spleen

gut

bone
marrow

Figure 8. The lymphoid system.
The organs of the lymphoid system are classified as primary or secondary. The primary organs are the sites where lymphocytes are produced. These are the bone marrow, thymus and the foetal liver. Lymphocytes produced in these migrate to the secondary organs, importantly, the spleen and lymph nodes, which are encapsulated organs, as well as the non-capsulated accumulations of lymphoid tissue throughout the body. Antigens become trapped in the lymph nodes as they filter the tissue lymph fluid passing through the lymphatic network during its passage from the periphery to the thoracic duct. There are approximately two million million lymphocytes in the healthy human adult. Of these, about half associate with the mucosal tissues indicating the importance of lymphocytes in providing protection against microorganisms that might gain entry to the body across mucous membranes.

LYMPHOCYTE DEVELOPMENT

The cells that recognize and react to antigens are lymphocytes. These cells are found throughout the body, in the blood and lymph fluid and are organized in lymphoid tissues known collectively as the lymphoid system (Figure 8).

In the developing foetus, cells migrate from the liver to the bone marrow to become the common precursors or stem cells

The cells of the immune system

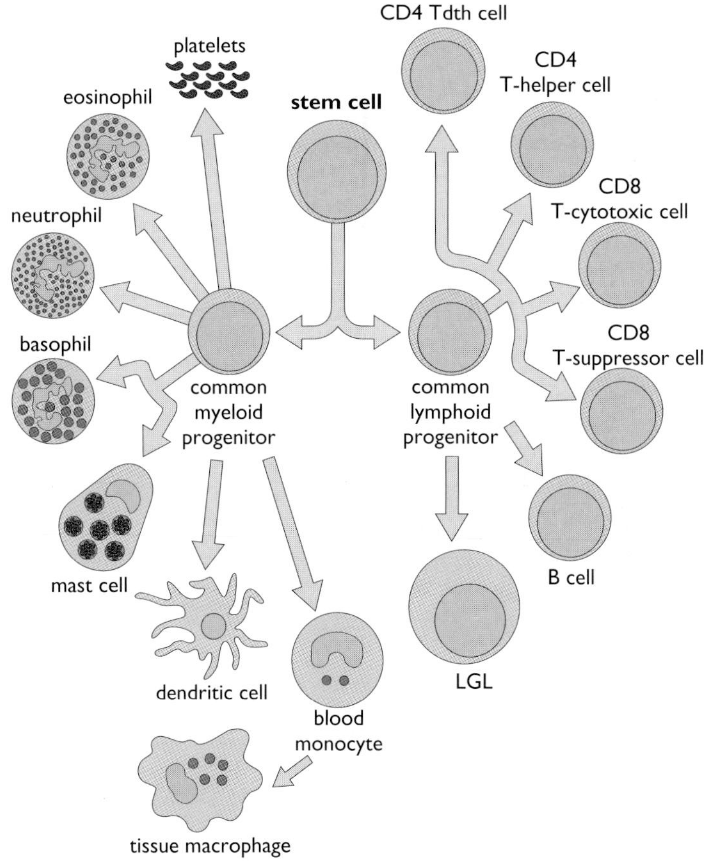

Figure 9. The cells of the immune system.
Two major categories of cells are derived from the common stem cell precursor: lymphoid and myeloid. Large granular lymphocytes (NK cells) are almost certainly lymphoid but their exact origin is uncertain. The roles played by these different types of cells are discussed in the text (cells not drawn to scale).

that are the source of lymphocytes and of all the other different cell types found in the blood. In the bone marrow, stem cells divide repeatedly and continuously producing many daughter cells. They are a self-generating source of all the cells that matter in effective immunity. As the cells divide they progressively become committed to a particular path of development, in other words their daughter cells differentiate to produce the various types of cells in the blood (Figure 9). The control of the production of all these cell types is a complex process but a number of *cytokines* are responsible for stimulating the growth of particular types of stem cell. This introduces you to this important group of proteins: cytokines are made by many different cells and are, by definition, molecular mediators that modify the function of other cells or the cells that made them in the first place. Cells

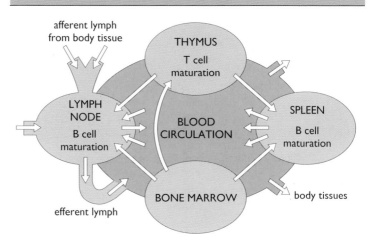

Lymphocyte development and circulation

Figure 10. Lymphocyte development and circulation.
In the adult, lymphoid stem cells in the bone marrow divide and produce lymphocyte precursor cells. These are destined to become two different types of lymphocyte and they all initially leave the marrow by the blood stream. Those that have passed through the thymus are called T cells, and in the thymus they complete their maturation to become antigen reactive cells. In the process of education in the thymus, they learn to recognize foreign antigens presented by MHC molecules. The other lymphocytes are B cells and they complete their maturation as they leave the marrow and go directly to the secondary lymphoid tissues. They do not go through an education comparable to that of T cells. Mature T cells and B cells circulate in the blood and migrate through body tissues whence they travel in the afferent lymph to lymph nodes, returning to the blood via the efferent vessels.

responsive to a particular cytokine have receptors on their cell membranes for that cytokine. As you will see later, other cytokines are also crucially important in regulating the activities of mature immune cells.

T Cell Maturation

Lymphocytes produced in the bone marrow enter the blood and circulate through the body. As illustrated in Figure 10, some of them pass through the thymus, re-enter the circulation and settle in the lymph nodes and spleen. These are called *T cells* and in their passage through the thymus they become subtly altered: there they acquire specificity which means that different lymphocytes become committed to recognizing different antigens. For example, a T cell may become specific for an antigen found only on the polio virus, and not be able to recognize those on any other virus.

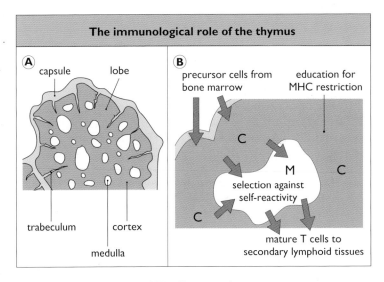

Figure 11. The thymus and T cell maturation.
(A) This is an illustration of a section of human thymus showing the main areas of the cortex C and medulla M. Note its lobulated structure contained within a capsule. Cells from the bone marrow first enter the cortex, from here they migrate to the medulla and later leave to colonise the secondary lymphoid tissues as indicated in (B). The educational process whereby T cells learn restriction by MHC molecules, and the destruction of self-reactive cells, both take place during this passage through the thymus. The interactions of maturing cells with epithelial reticular cells and macrophages are thought to be involved in this education and selection processes.

We have recently learned much more about the fascinating process of T cell maturation in the thymus (Figure 11). As we have said before, most of the cells that enter the thymus die there in a process designed to eliminate those cells with a tendency to react in a damaging way with self antigens. However, when mature T cells react outside the thymus with foreign antigens, they do so by recognizing them in association with some self molecules on other cells that are said to present the antigen to the T cells. Thus, interestingly, the ability of T cells to recognize 'foreignness' also requires that the cells interact with and recognize some particular self molecules. The self molecules that are important in this are cell surface proteins known as *major histocompatibility complex* (MHC) molecules (there are two types important in this context, class I and class II), and T cells acquire the capacity to recognize these particular self molecules in a certain way in the thymus. Thymus education involves a process in which cells that react too strongly or too weakly with self MHC molecules are exterminated; those that survive then mature and recognize foreign antigens together with MHC molecules. Furthermore, the MHC molecules in the thymus also present small fragments of degraded, or processed, peptides of many other self proteins to the developing T cells; any T cells with the potential to respond to these are also exterminated. In this way self-reactive, or autoreactive, T cells that could be harmful are destroyed.

T cells have recognition molecules known as *T cell receptors* (TCR) on their cell surface which react with antigen. Each T cell has a slightly different version of the TCR, and hence a slightly different specificity. We should emphasize that the great diversity of these T cells, the so-called T cell repertoire, is created by natural mechanisms without the involvement of the foreign antigens against which the T cells are later capable of responding. So the immune system is designed to develop its *immunocompetence* without outside influence.

B Cell Maturation
Other lymphocytes do not pass through the thymus but settle directly in the secondary lymphoid tissues – the lymph nodes and the spleen. These are called *B cells*, and as they mature they do not go through the highly selective processes to which T cells are subjected. Although potentially autoreactive B cells are eliminated during development, many survive and become part of the normal make up of the healthy adult. It is likely that B cells essentially complete their maturation in the bone marrow before entering the secondary lymphoid tissues. With B cells, as with T cells, this early development or maturation happens quite

independently of exposure to foreign antigens. B cells carry (or are said to express) on their surface antibody molecules which act as their receptors for antigen. The antibody receptors on each antigen-reactive B cell are specific for one antigen only. Although antibodies are different from TCR molecules, both are receptors for antigen and they have, as will be explained, some common structural features.

The electron photomicrographs of major different lymphocyte types in Figure 12 summarize their gross structural differences and show the effects of activation on them.

LYMPHOCYTE ACTIVATION

T cells and B cells constitute the two important sets of lymphocytes that respond to antigens. Although they are different in their origins and in the ways they react with antigen, each set has a repertoire of specificities from which particular members can be selected to respond specifically to individual antigens. The size of each repertoire is large and reflects the fact that we need to be able to respond to an enormous number of foreign antigens. It is impossible to calculate accurately how many different antigens there are, but it is certainly greater than one million million! As the average adult human has around two million million lymphocytes, it is likely that we have a few lymphocytes capable of responding to any antigen we are likely to encounter. On their own, these cells are numerically insufficient to deal effectively with this sort of challenge, so mechanisms exist that permit the most useful cells to increase their numbers by multiplying when needed.

B Cell Activation

When a B cell is exposed to an antigen it differentiates from an antigen-reactive B cell (Figure 12A) into either an antibody secreting cell – which becomes a *plasma cell* (Figure 12C) – or a memory cell. The combination of antigen with the antibody receptor on the cell surface of the B cell generates signals inside the cell that switch on its antibody-producing machinery. In the first stage the cell becomes activated (Figure 12B), it then multiplies and differentiates to form a *clone* of daughter cells which start secreting antibody of the same type as that expressed originally on the surface of the parent cell. This antibody combines with the antigen, initiating a chain of events leading to the destruction or neutralization of the antigen. Most of the daughter cells die after a few weeks. A proportion of them, however, do not make antibody to any great extent but recirculate in the body and may persist for many years as memory cells. If they are **23**

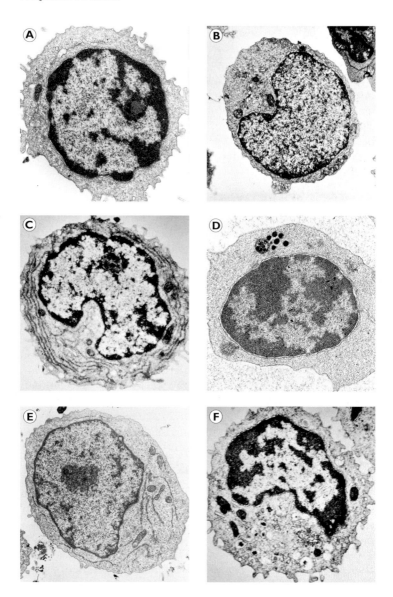

Figure 12. The structure of lymphocytes
Transmission electron micrographs showing the typical structure of lymphocytes.
(A) Resting B cell. (B) B cell blast shortly after activation with antigen. (C) Plasma
cell, the end cell derived from a B cell blast that secretes large amounts of
antibody for a few days before it dies. (D) Resting T cell. (E) T cell blast after
activation with antigen. Such cells typically produce cytokines, some become
cytotoxic. (F) A large granular lymphocyte (LGL), or NK, cell that is cytotoxic
(see also Figure 7). (Not to scale – cells enlarge upon activation.)

subsequently exposed again to the same antigen they rapidly become activated and make more antibody. In this way secondary immune responses occur (Figure 13). The same antibody is produced again but at a faster rate than in the primary response which followed the first exposure to the antigen. This happens because more antigen-reactive cells exist as a result of clonal expansion and because they go through fewer divisions before they secrete antibody. These enhanced specific secondary responses are said to demonstrate immunological memory.

Clonal expansion provides a highly efficient way to produce large amounts of antibody without the necessity of initially possessing large numbers of each specific lymphocyte. The importance of this can be appreciated when it is realized that after immunization there may be thousands of cells making the same antibody and that the immune system has the potential to make millions of different antibodies.

T Cell Activation

T cells (Figure 12D) do not make antibodies or secrete special forms of their antigen receptor molecules. Instead, after reacting with antigen they go through similar stages of activation, growth and differentiation and secrete a variety of cytokines (Figure 12E). These mediators are especially important in regulating the function of other lymphocytes. It is recognized that there are different types, or sub-sets, of T cells that serve different functions by virtue of the different cytokines they produce. Furthermore, T cells express particular accessory molecules on their cell surface that are important to their function, but which incidentally are very useful to immunologists as an aid to identify and classify them. Thus, *T-helper cells* (also known as TH2 cells) express structures known as CD4 molecules on their surface. T-helper cells are important in helping B cells make antibody responses by synthesizing and secreting cytokines that promote the activation, growth and differentiation of B cells. Other cells, also known as *T-suppressor cells*, express CD8 molecules on their surface, and counterbalance the effects of T cell help and suppress immune responses. Therefore, T cells control the activity of each other and other cells of the immune system through making cytokines.

The measurement of T cells expressing either CD4 or CD8 has become clinically important as changes in the natural balance between helper and suppressor cells may be an indication of changes in the healthy functioning of the immune system. Thus in AIDS, for example, the $CD8^+$ population dominates the cells in the peripheral blood, indicating that immune function is compromised. **25**

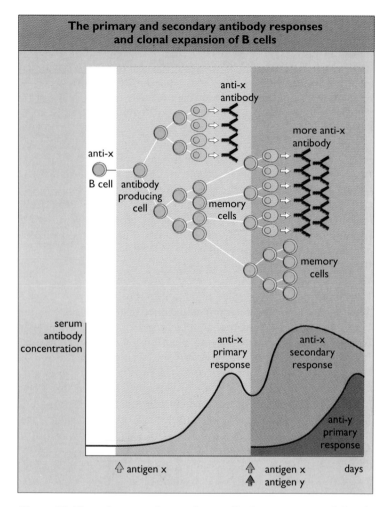

The primary and secondary antibody responses and clonal expansion of B cells

Figure 13. The primary and secondary antibody responses and clonal expansion of B cells.

In a typical demonstration of primary and secondary responses the concentration of serum antibody against antigen x is assayed on successive days. The antigen stimulates B cells to grow and differentiate into antibody-producing cells called plasma cells. Antibody concentration reaches a peak and declines as plasma cells die. This is known as the primary response. A small proportion of antigen-stimulated B cells do not turn into plasma cells but survive as memory cells. When the same antigen is encountered on a second (or subsequent) occasion, antibody is produced more rapidly and in greater quantity as a result of the clonal expansion that followed the first contact with antigen. This is the secondary response and it is specific for antigen x: a different antigen (y) injected at the same time produces only a primary response by activating anti-y cells (not illustrated).

However, not all T cells are regulatory. Some of the CD8$^+$ cells can kill other cells and are known as *T-cytotoxic cells*. They are primarily responsible for destroying cells of the body that have been infected with viruses. Although the infected cell is destroyed by the cytotoxic process, this is a relatively small price to pay since the virus cannot then replicate. Finally, some CD4$^+$ T cells are important in certain types of hypersensitivity reactions. These are known as Tdth cells or TH1 cells (dth means *delayed-type hypersensitivity*) and they are involved in cell-mediated immune responses such as the destruction of intracellular bacteria, some types of delayed hypersensitivities, autoimmune diseases and the rejection of organ transplants. All these are discussed later. Although the T cells that help B cells make antibodies (TH2) and the T cells that are involved in delayed-type hypersensitivity (Tdth) all have CD4 molecules, they differ from each other in the types of cytokines that they make. It is these that enable them to do different things.

Large Granular Lymphocytes

There is a third population of lymphocytes that have two peculiar properties. They lack antibody or T cell receptor molecules on their surface and they contain many granules of pharmacologically active substances (Figure 12F). These large granular lymphocytes are cytotoxic and are probably important, as we discussed earlier, in non-specific immunity to tumour cells, virus-infected cells and in regulating production of blood cells in the bone marrow. They are also known as NK cells.

Cytokines

These have been mentioned in several different contexts and some of the more important examples are listed in Table 3. Immune cells usually make more than one cytokine when activated. Each individual cytokine can have several different functions according to which cell(s) it binds to. In all cases a cell can only respond to a cytokine if it expresses the appropriate receptor; when the cytokine binds to this a signal is transmitted into the cell that will activate particular genes thereby changing the activity of the cell. We must stress the importance of various cytokines in controlling the activity of lymphocytes themselves. Thus, the activation of both T cells and B cells is critically dependent upon receiving signals delivered by appropriate cytokines binding to receptors on their cell membranes.

We refer to the multi-functional effects of cytokines as pleiotropy, literally meaning many different effects. It is easiest to imagine these important molecules working in a network that **27**

Cytokines with important immune functions		
Cytokine	Origin	Major effects
Lymphocyte activation		
IL-1	Antigen-presenting cells	Initial activation of T cells
IL-2	Activated TH1 T cells	Growth of T cells
IFN-γ	Activated TH1 T cells	Inhibits effect of IL-4 on B cells
IL-4	Activated TH2 T cells	Activation and differentiation of B cells
IL-10	Activated TH2 T cells	Suppression of TH1 T cells
TGF-β	Various cells	Suppression of TH1 T cells
Local inflammation		
IL-1	Various cells	Activation of neutrophils
IL-2	Activated T cells	Chemotaxis and activation of macrophages
Colony-stimulating factors (various)	Various cells	Growth and activation of phagocytic cells
IFN-γ	T cells	Phagocyte activation
TNF	Monocytes, lymphocytes	Neutrophil activation
Chemokines (including IL-8)	Various cells	Attract cells to sites of inflammation
Systemic inflammation		
IL-1 and IL-6	Many cells	Stimulates bone marrow Acute phase protein synthesis Fever induction
TNF		Fever induction Acute phase protein production

Table 3. Cytokines with important immune functions.
It is impossible in simplifying the cytokines to give a precise account. This is because (a) different cytokines share effects and so may replace each other in their actions (this is called redundancy), (b) individual cytokines have many properties (this is called pleiotropy), (c) a particular cytokine may be made by several different cells, and (d) cytokines act synergistically or antagonistically with each other.

regulates and controls both immune cells and also many other cells of the body: this is one way of understanding how the immune system interacts with other physiological systems and how they are mutually dependent on each other.

Be aware that the nomenclature of cytokines is a little complicated: *lymphokines* and monokines, which have historically older names, are all cytokines; the *interleukins* are cytokines made by leucocytes that affect primarily other leucocytes, the *chemokines* are especially involved in initiating inflammation. The word cytokine itself is used by some to refer only to molecules that affect immune function; others give it a more general meaning and we favour this use of the word.

Major Histocompatibility Complex (MHC) Molecules

All cells of the body in mammals, and probably in all other vertebrates as well, have a set of proteins in their membranes which are products of genes of the MHC. These membrane molecules are of two types, known as class I and class II MHC molecules. They regulate T cell activity in such a way that the T cells only recognize foreign antigens when they are associated with the MHC molecules themselves. The MHC, which is known as the *HLA system* in man, is a highly *polymorphic* genetic system: it is extremely unlikely to find two unrelated individuals with the same collection of MHC products. Because the MHC varies so much between different individuals, it follows that when tissues or organs are transplanted the MHC molecules in them act as *transplantation antigens* and activate the recipient's lymphocytes which can then destroy the graft.

The Many Functions of Lymphocytes

The lymphocytes of the body are dedicated to performing certain tasks which are initiated by immunologically specific recognition events: some make antibodies, some destroy virus-infected cells, and some regulate the activity of other cell types. An immune response involves some or all of these populations which interact and cooperate with each other in a complex way to deal with the particular antigenic challenge. The type of response varies with the nature of the antigen, its dose and the route by which it enters the body. It also depends on previous exposure to the same antigen and on many constitutional factors in the host itself. Lymphocytes do not, however, operate in isolation but they depend upon each other and other cell types both in order to be activated and also to express their immunological activities.

PHAGOCYTES AND ANTIGEN-PRESENTING CELLS

Macrophages and PMNs are actively phagocytic and can ingest and destroy bacteria, viruses, etc. This process is greatly enhanced if the particles are coated, or *opsonized*, with specific antibodies and further enhanced by certain components of the complement system (Figure 14).

Although antigens activate lymphocytes, very few antigens appear to bind directly to antigen-reactive T cells or B cells. Instead they are usually presented to the lymphocytes on the surface of other cells known collectively as *antigen-presenting cells* (APCs) (Figure 15). One important group of APCs are *dendritic cells* which are widely distributed in the body. They appear to trap antigens, thereby concentrating them and preventing their spread, and then initiate local immune responses.

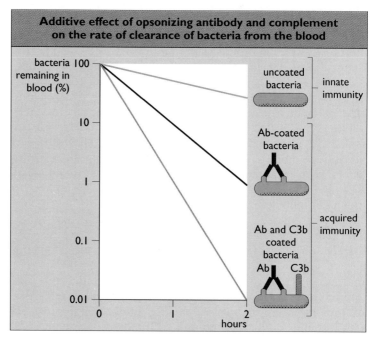

Figure 14. Effect of opsonizing antibody and complement on the rate of clearance of bacteria from the blood.
Uncoated bacteria are processed by the natural immune system and as a result they are cleared from the blood relatively slowly. An antibody coating on the surface of the bacteria facilitates their attachment to phagocytes which possess receptors for the Fc part of the antibody. The bacteria are cleared more rapidly as a consequence. Phagocytes also possess receptors for the complement component C3b. If the bacteria also become coated with C3b, then phagocytic attachment and bacterial clearance will be further enhanced.

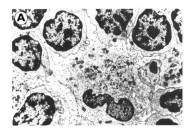
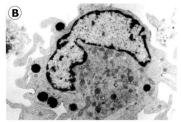

Figure 15. Antigen-presenting cells.
(A) Electron micrograph of an interdigitating cell in the T cell area of a lymph node. The cell at the centre has an enormous surface area in which antigen is presented to the surrounding T cells. (B) Dendritic cells are the mobile precursors of interdigitating cells and are found throughout the body. This one was isolated from the joint fluid of a patient with arthritis and it illustrates the great number of dendritic processes that create the large surface area of the cell. This cell expresses MHC class II molecules on its surface. Courtesy of Stella Knight and Patsy Fryer.

Dendritic Cells

Dendritic cells in lymph nodes and the spleen trap antigen circulating in the lymph and blood and present it to the resident lymphocytes. Similarly, in non-lymphoid tissues, dendritic cells trap antigen and then migrate themselves to the lymphoid tissues thus carrying antigen to the cells capable of reacting to it. The architecture of the lymph nodes and spleen is such that APCs and reactive lymphocytes are in close contact in the same micro-environment. A lymph node under antigenic stimulation contains proliferating cells (clonal expansion) that form lymphoid follicles containing foci, known as *germinal centres*, of B cells that make specific antibody, T cells and dendritic cells. Germinal centres are especially important in generating memory B cells. In other areas of the node, T cells are seen to proliferate and will usually include T-helper and T-cytotoxic cells and Tdth cells (Figure 16). Comparable changes occur in the spleen when antigen stimulates it (Figure 17). The types of T cells seen in stimulated lymphoid tissues vary with the nature of the antigenic stimulus and with the duration of the immune response.

Macrophages

These can also present antigens to lymphocytes but they probably do this less effectively than dendritic cells. The main role of the macrophage is to 'eat' and destroy, whereas the role of dendritic cells, which are not phagocytic like macrophages, is to concentrate antigens on their surface membranes (which may have an enormous surface area), to make them accessible to lymphocytes.   31

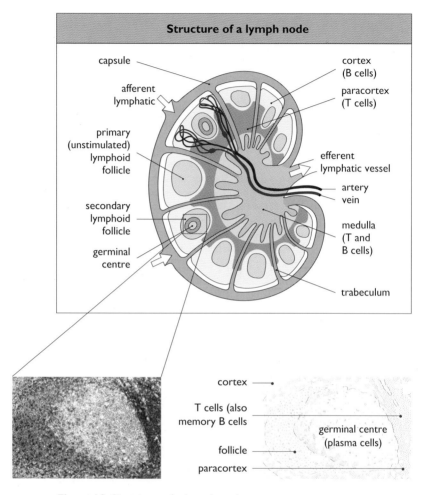

Figure 16. Structure of a lymph node.
The organ consists of a cortex, paracortex and medulla and is enclosed by a capsule. Lymphocytes and antigens pass into the node through the afferent lymphatics. The lymph (fluid and lymphocytes) drains through the node and passes out of the medulla through the efferent lymphatic vessel. The cortex contains B cells aggregated into primary follicles; following stimulation by antigen these become secondary follicles and develop foci of active proliferation (germinal centres). Cells in the follicles are in intimate contact with antigen-presenting dendritic cells. The paracortex contains T cells, and the medulla contains both T and B cells. Each node has its own blood supply by which lymphocytes can also enter. Micrograph courtesy of Peter Amlot.

The structure of the spleen

tributary of
splenic vein

trabecular
tissue

splenic vein
splenic artery

trabeculum
venous sinuses
red pulp
PALS
(white pulp)
lobular vein
lobular artery

to splenic vein
from splenic artery

red
pulp

marginal zone
follicular artery
germinal centre
T-dependent area

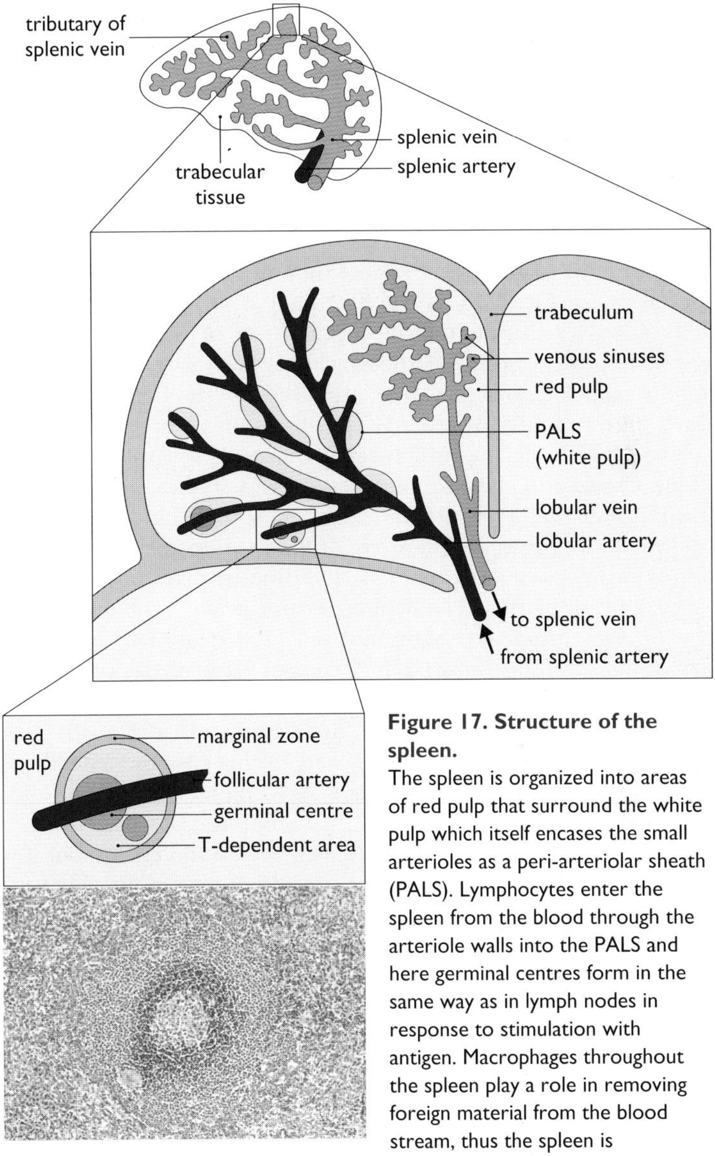

Figure 17. Structure of the spleen.
The spleen is organized into areas of red pulp that surround the white pulp which itself encases the small arterioles as a peri-arteriolar sheath (PALS). Lymphocytes enter the spleen from the blood through the arteriole walls into the PALS and here germinal centres form in the same way as in lymph nodes in response to stimulation with antigen. Macrophages throughout the spleen play a role in removing foreign material from the blood stream, thus the spleen is concerned with providing protection mostly against blood-borne infection and the lymph nodes with protection against infection in the tissues.

33

B Cells

During antibody responses, activated B cells can also act as very efficient presenting cells. In this role they are probably by far the most important cell type for amplifying their own secondary antibody responses. They present antigen to T-helper cells that in turn make cytokines that stimulate the B cells to further differentiate and produce antibody. In contrast, when the numbers of specific B cells are low at the start of a primary immune response, dendritic cells are the more important presenters of antigen to T-helper cells.

Mechanisms of Antigen Processing and Presentation

Before it is presented to a T cell, antigen is processed by an APC. This involves the enzymatic degradation of the antigen into small peptides. Some of these, if they have the right sort of amino acid sequence, become anchored to class I (peptides of 8 or 9 amino acids) or class II (peptides of 12 or more amino acids) MHC molecules which act as receptors for processed peptides. Class I and class II molecules are very similar, but not identical in their overall structure (see later) so they bind peptides in slightly different ways. There are at least two major pathways for antigen processing (Figure 18). The first involves proteins that are taken up by the APC by phagocytosis or some other form of endocytosis (often receptor-mediated) and degraded within the lysosomal compartment. The peptides from these ultimately associate with class II MHC molecules and cycle to the cell surface. The second pathway is dedicated to dealing with proteins synthesized within the cell, and in this case their degradation peptides associate with class I MHC molecules in the Golgi system before transport to the cell membrane. Proteins synthesized in the cell can also associate with class II molecules, but it is not clear where this actually happens, although it is possible they need first to reach the cell membrane to enter the endocytic pathway. The class I pathway is especially important for presentation of virus proteins which are, of course, synthesized in the host cells.

Restriction of T Cell Activation

The two different pathways are concerned with the activation of different types of T cells. Thus, the MHC class II endocytic pathway is concerned with CD4$^+$ T cells, such as T-helper and Tdth cells, and the MHC class I Golgi pathway with T-cytotoxic CD8$^+$ cells. In this way, T cells with different surface accessory molecules (CD4 or CD8) are restricted to being activated by one or other class of MHC molecule and by antigens processed in different ways. So you

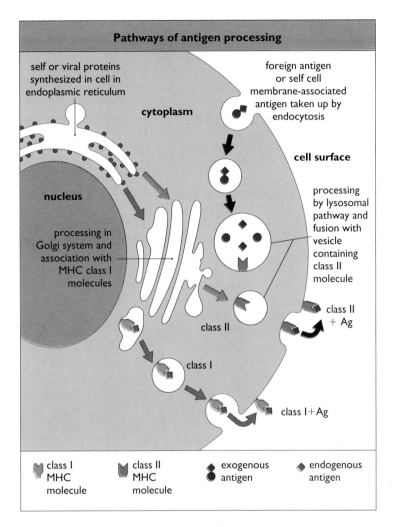

Figure 18. Pathways of antigen processing.
The two main pathways of processing protein antigens for presentation to T cells. Proteins made inside the cell, and this includes viral proteins, may be degraded and their peptides bound by MHC class I molecules in the Golgi system and transported to the cell membrane where they are then presented to CD8[+] T cells The other route involves the endocytosis of proteins from outside the cell. These are degraded in endosomal vesicles and bound by MHC class II molecules which cycle to the cell membrane where the peptides are presented to CD4[+] T cells. The endosomal pathway is used for processing both foreign proteins and self proteins that associate with the cell membrane. Although class II molecules, whilst in the Golgi system, usually bind a so-called invariant chain polypeptide that prevents them binding degraded self peptides, it is possible that some self peptides do associate with them at this stage.

can see that $CD4^+$ T-helper cells are concerned especially with responses against external or exogenous antigens, whereas $CD8^+$ T-cytotoxic cells are concerned with responses against antigens that are behaving as self molecules by virtue of being synthesized inside cells of the body. It is interesting and important to realize that MHC class I molecules are normally present upon all nucleated cells, which means that anti-viral immune reactions can be generated to deal with infection anywhere in the body. On the other hand, class II molecules are limited to various types of antigen-presenting cells under normal healthy conditions, and so $CD4^+$ T-helper cells are activated by antigens in more restricted circumstances than $CD8^+$ cells simply by virtue of the way in which class I and class II molecules are expressed in different places.

Together, these mechanisms ensure that T cells are activated only in the right place, at the right time and in response to processed antigen. This last point emphasizes the basic difference in antigen recognition by T cells and B cells. In general, B cells respond to intact proteins and T cells respond to processed or degraded proteins. We should note that activated B cells are good presenting cells because firstly their surface antibody acts as a receptor for antigen which is then endocytosed, and secondly they express quite large amounts of MHC class II molecules that can present the peptides from the processed antigen. A little thought will now tell you that B cells and T cells are likely to recognize different parts of the same protein antigen molecule, and indeed this is the case. We refer to the small parts of an antigen that are recognized by the TCR or antibody as *epitopes*. It will become apparent later that understanding which epitopes of an antigen can induce protective immunity to infectious agents is very valuable in designing vaccines to protect against disease.

Cell Cooperation

The important cell interactions involved in the activation of T cells and B cells are summarized in Figure 19. With the exception of a few antibody responses it appears that all immune responses depend upon T cells. In general, antigens must be presented by an appropriate cell and the generation of so-called effector plasma cells and T-cytotoxic cells is amplified by T-helper cells and restrained by Tdth and T-suppressor cells. We have only an incomplete picture of the molecular events of cell interaction but we do know that antigen, MHC molecules, accessory molecules and cytokines are very important in effective co-operation between immune cells.

The interactions of cells involved in immune responses

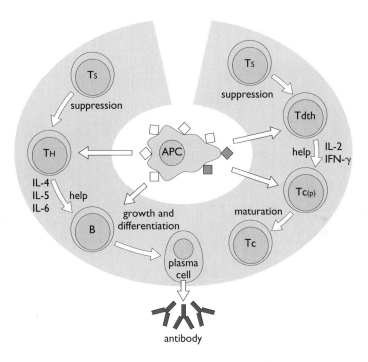

Figure 19. The interactions of cells involved in immune responses.
The antigen-presenting cell (APC) at the centre varies according to the type of
cell to which antigen is presented. B cells respond initially to an intact antigen
on an APC and are helped by CD4$^+$ T-helper (TH) cells that in turn respond to
processed antigen presented in association with MHC class II molecules on
APCs. In secondary immune responses, the B cells themselves may take on the
function of APCs, presenting antigen to T-helper cells that then back-stimulate
the B cells. The activation of CD8$^+$ T-cytotoxic cell precursors (Tc(p)) involves
the presentation of processed antigens, this time in association with MHC class
I molecules, and their activation may also be helped by another population of
CD4$^+$ T-helper cells that through cytokine production, cause delayed-type
hypersensitivity (Tdth cells). In both the B cell and T-helper/T-cytotoxic arms
of the response illustrated, some control is exerted by suppressive CD8$^+$ T-
suppressor cells (Ts). Their activation may not necessarily depend upon
presentation of processed antigen in association with MHC molecules. The two
types of CD4$^+$ cells also interact to regulate each other's activities. At all
stages, the interaction between cells depends not only upon processed antigen
plus MHC but also upon various cytokines, the most important of which are
indicated. In addition, the physical interaction between cells involves adhesion
molecule interactions.

37

OTHER CELLS INVOLVED IN IMMUNE RESPONSES

Particular types of immune responses involve certain other cells as illustrated in Figure 20. These include *mast cells, basophils, eosinophils,* natural killer cells and lymphokine activated killer (LAK) cells.

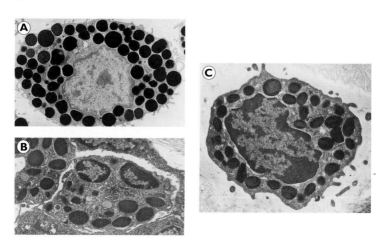

Figure 20. Mast cells, basophils and eosinophils.
These cells are related to neutrophils but have specialized functions: the mast cell (A) and basophil (B) depend upon passively absorbed IgE antibodies and have important roles in immediate type allergic reactions exemplified by asthma and hay fever and anti-parasite immunity. The eosinophil (C) likewise depends upon IgE and some types of IgG antibodies to exert its cytotoxic functions that are important in the same types of immune responses. All the cells contain granules of pharmacological mediators that become activated upon triggering through cell membrane receptors: they cause local inflammatory reactions.

Mast Cells and Basophils

Tissue mast cells contain granules of pharmacologically active substances. They have antibodies of the IgE class (see later) fixed on their surface membranes and when these bind specific antigens the cells are triggered to degranulate releasing the substances in the granules which promote local inflammatory reactions leading to the accumulation of PMNs, monocytes, and lymphocytes, thus bringing to a local site the cells best able to deal with the antigen and destroy it. Quite a large number of mast cells are associated with the mucosal tissues. They are particularly important in responses to inhaled antigens such as pollens and house dust that cause the *hay fever* type of allergy which affects the lungs, and in dealing with infection by certain parasitic worms that infest the gut.

Basophilic polymorphonuclear leucocytes, known as basophils (and related to neutrophils), contain similar granules and function in much the same was as mast cells.

Eosinophils

Eosinophils are also closely related to neutrophils and are specialized cells important in the extracellular killing of parasites too large to be phagocytosed by other cells. For this they depend upon IgG and IgE antibodies coating the parasite. Extracellular killing is not a property restricted to eosinophils. Monocytes, macrophages and some lymphocytes can kill microorganisms coated with antibodies and when expressing this activity these cells are known collectively as killer or *K cells*. Natural killer cells mentioned before also exhibit this property of extracellular killing, but independently of specific antibody.

Lymphokine Activated Killer (LAK) Cells

Another group of cells attracting the attention of scientists are *lymphocyte activated killer*, or LAK cells. These can be created intentionally by treating lymphocytes with cytokines *in vitro*. This process activates the cells and makes them capable of killing some tumour cells. Accordingly, they may become valuable in treating certain forms of cancer when given back to the patient.

ANTIGEN RECEPTOR MOLECULES

The cells of the immune system respond selectively to antigens because they have receptors for them. As emphasized earlier, each lymphocyte has a unique specificity acquired during its maturation, and the reason for this is that it has a receptor of slightly different structure from that of any other cell. In biochemical terms, it is the particular sequence of the amino acids making up each receptor that gives it its functional specificity through imparting to it a unique three-dimensional structure. There are three types or groups of molecules that act as antigen receptors. Each member of each group differs only slightly from the others in the group: they are said to be highly polymorphic.

The Immunoglobulin Superfamily

Antibodies, which belong to the group of proteins called *immunoglobulins*, act as receptors for antigen on B cells. These were the first antigen-binding molecules to be discovered. However, the TCR molecules of T cells and the MHC molecules that present antigen share with antibodies the common property of binding or recognizing antigen. **39**

Advances in protein chemistry and molecular genetics have allowed scientists to look carefully at these receptors and they have found that their shared function is because they also share many detailed structural and genetic features. In fact, the similarities between the different parts (domains) of the molecules are so compelling that it is believed that they all evolved from a primordial gene that diversified and duplicated to give the great range of receptor molecules seen today in higher vertebrates. Acknowledging their historical primacy, antibodies are classified, together with TCR and MHC molecules (and their genes), as members of the immunoglobulin superfamily.

The immunoglobulin supergene family	
Category	Members
Antigen receptors	Antibody/immunoglobulin T cell receptor α/β, γ/δ and CD3 MHC molecules class I and II

Molecules that regulate lymphocytes	CD2 (all T cells)
	CD4 (helper T cells)
	CD8 (cytotoxic T cells)
	Leucocyte functional antigen-3
	  (LFA-3), intracellular adhesion
	  molecule-1 (ICAM-1)

Receptors that bind constant parts of immunoglobulins	Immunoglobulin Fc receptors (various) Poly Ig receptor on epithelial cells
Neural molecules	Thy-1, OX2, neural cell adhesion molecule (NCAM), contactin

Receptors for growth factors/cytokines	PDGF receptor, CSF-1 receptor,
	  FGF receptor, IL-1 receptor,
	  IL-6 receptor, GCSF receptor

Receptors for viruses	HIV-1 (CD4), rhinovirus (ICAM-1), poliovirus receptor
Antigens on tumour cells	Carcinoembryonic antigen (CEA), NCA, gp-70, MUC 18

Table 4. The immunoglobulin supergene family.
This is a simplified list to give an indication of the range of biological activities associated with molecules that, because of their structural similarities, are members of the immunoglobulin superfamily. Some molecules, such as ICAM-1 and CD4, appear more than once because they have more than one known function. Note that all functions involve recognition events at the cell membrane.

This superfamily also includes several hundred other members, some of which are listed in Table 4. All these molecules are concerned with recognition and interaction events between cells. The way to think of the polymorphic antigen receptors of the immune system is as specialized descendents of molecules that had a role in helping cells recognize each other. You will note that some molecules in the list have already been mentioned in the context of T cell activity (CD4 and CD8) and the adhesion of phagocytic cells to vascular endothelial cells (CD18). Others, such as some complement receptors, we will meet later on.

In the sections that follow we will describe in more detail the structure of the antigen receptors so that you may understand more clearly how they function. Each is shown in simplified form in Figure 21 which is designed to emphasize their similarities. One of the impressive features of the MHC, TCR and antibody systems is that they each have the same structure in all vertebrates, which is what you would expect from an evolutionary point of view for important molecules that have sophisticated structures for subtle functions. What follows concentrates upon the systems in humans, but the general principles apply to the antigen receptors in all mammals.

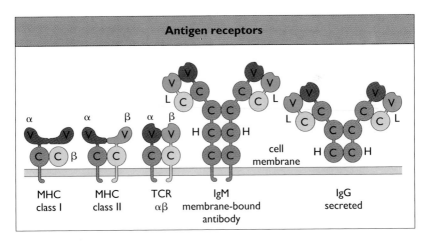

Figure 21. Antigen receptors.
There are three types of receptors for antigen: the MHC molecules, the TCR molecules and antibodies or immunoglobulins. All share structural features that show they have evolved from a common ancestor molecule. Each is characterized by domains that are either constant (C) or variable (V) between all molecules of that type, and because of their similarity to immunoglobulins in this regard they are thought of collectively as members of the immunoglobulin superfamily.

THE MAJOR HISTOCOMPATIBILITY COMPLEX

MHC molecules of both classes have quite similar overall structures and are located in the membranes of cells presenting their antigen binding sites to the outside environment. The degraded antigen peptides that are bound by the MHC molecules sit in a cleft on the top of the molecule that is most easily demonstrated in the picture (Figure 22) derived from an X-ray crystallographic analysis of an HLA molecule. The different sequences of amino acids in the different HLA molecules located in the areas of the flat floor and helical sides of the binding cleft determine which antigen peptides can be bound. In fact, HLA molecules are not particularly fastidious about which peptides they bind, so in comparison with antibodies, for example, they exhibit a rather low specificity for antigen.

Class I and Class II Genes

The genetic organization of the MHC is very complex. A simplified version of the human HLA system is shown in Figure 23. For each of the class I genes there are many different alternative versions, or *alleles*, as shown. By conventional tissue typing we know of at least 26 for the A gene, 35 for the B gene and 14 for the C gene. Each individual has two chromosomes carrying these genes and so has up to, but no more than, six different class I gene alleles. Hence, although class I molecules (the direct protein products of the genes) are expressed on all cells, there will not be more than six different versions of the class I molecules

Figure 22. MHC molecules and processed antigens.
This model of an MHC class I molecule was derived from X-ray diffraction studies of a crystal of pure HLA-B27 molecules solubilized from the surface of lymphocytes. The molecule has a characteristic structure in which the C domains of the large α and small β (actually β_2-microglobulin) polypeptide chains pack close to the cell membrane, and the two V domains (α_1 and α_2) of the α chain are folded in a unique way to create a binding site for the processed antigen peptide. The molecule is seen from the side in (A) and its binding site from above in (B). The peptide sits in the binding site groove like a hot dog in a bun. The T cell receptor interacts with both the peptide and the helical parts of the MHC molecule as shown in Figure 24. The structure of MHC class II molecules is very similar to this although the two polypeptides are of more nearly equal size with the α and the β chains each contributing a V domain to the peptide binding site. The great polymorphism of these molecules is represented by subtle variations in the amino acid sequences of the helical structures around the binding site and of the flat parallel strands in the floor of the binding site. These dictate the sequences of the processed peptides that can be bound by any particular MHC molecule. In this illustration, B is 0.5 $\times$ size of A.

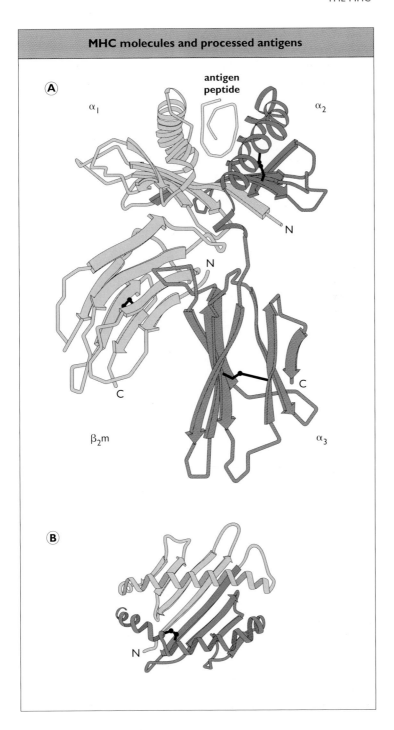

MHC molecules and processed antigens

Ⓐ

α₁

antigen
peptide

α₂

N

N

C

C

β₂m

α₃

Ⓑ

N

present. Similarly, there are many different alleles for each class II gene and these are also shown in Figure 23. Class II genes are not expressed in every cell, but on those cells that do express them, there will be no more that six different versions of the class II molecules, because there are three different genes and two chromosomes coding them.

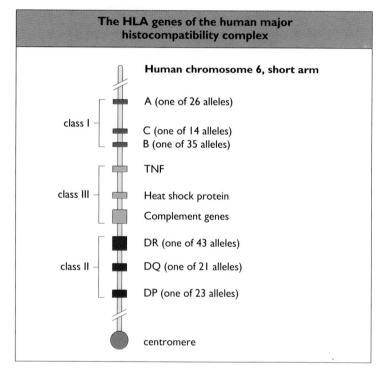

The HLA genes of the human major histocompatibility complex

Human chromosome 6, short arm

class I
- A (one of 26 alleles)
- C (one of 14 alleles)
- B (one of 35 alleles)

class III
- TNF
- Heat shock protein
- Complement genes

class II
- DR (one of 43 alleles)
- DQ (one of 21 alleles)
- DP (one of 23 alleles)

centromere

Figure 23. The HLA genes of the MHC.
This shows the way the HLA genes are arranged on chromosome 6 in humans. The features of this MHC are also seen in the MHCs of other animals. Note how the class I genes are all close together, likewise the class II and class III genes. Each individual inherits two sets of these genes, one from the mother and one from the father, and so has two chromosomes coding MHC genes. As all the genes can be expressed, we each have up to six different class I and six different class II molecules on the surfaces of our cells. All the class I and II genes are extremely polymorphic which means that the chances of finding two unrelated individuals with the same MHC genes is vanishingly small. The numbers of alleles shown are certainly underestimates of the real numbers. Notice that the so-called class III genes code for molecules such as those of the complement system and the cytokine TNF which, although they are relatively non-polymorphic and have no specificity for antigen, are important immunologically.

Polymorphism

The polymorphism of the HLA system is very large at the level of the human population, although in each individual a small number of alleles code for an equally limited number of molecules. However, because there can be any one of each of the possible alleles at each respective gene position, you will realize that two unrelated individuals are extremely unlikely to have the same HLA make up. To understand how diverse we all are in our HLA genes, do the following exercise. Calculate how many potentially different combinations of A, B, C, DR, DP and DQ alleles there are by multiplying together all the different alleles possible at each gene. Each possible permutation is called a *haplotype*, and each individual has two different haplotypes (making the genotype), so the number of different haplotype pairings – a measure of our population diversity – is the square of the number of haplotypes!

Class III Genes

The part of the chromosome that carries the HLA genes also has a number of other genes (also known as MHC class III genes) of particular interest to immunologists. These include genes for tumour necrosis factors (TNF-α and TNF-β) which are important cytokines, and for some components of the complement system. The fact that the same genes are also found in the MHC of other species suggests that their association with the class I and II genes is no accident, but at the moment we can only guess at its significance. However, we do know that the MHC genes include several that code for proteins that are very important in the transport, degradation and protection of proteins inside the cell. Their main roles may well be in protecting proteins from degradation whilst they are being assembled, and also to protect proteins against various forms of shock, including heat which will denature proteins. The same proteins seem to have a role in the antigen processing described earlier.

It is widely thought that the whole MHC represents a collection of genes that have the purpose to produce the machinery for protein handling inside the cell.

THE T CELL RECEPTOR (TCR)

The TCR is a complex collection of polypeptides, of which two particular polypeptide chains give it antigen specificity. The most common combination is an α and β chain. There is another version that contains γ and δ chains. Like all other antigen receptors, these molecules reside in the cell membrane and present their antigen receptor site to the outside (see Figure 21).

45

We explained earlier that T cells require antigenic peptides to be presented by an MHC molecule to the TCR. Thus, the TCR interacts with both the antigen peptide and either a class I or class II MHC molecule. The αβ chain pair alone is not enough for a functional receptor, and these polypeptides associate with other peptides on the T cell surface that make up the CD3 molecule – another product of the immunoglobulin supergene family. It is the CD3 part of the complex that transmits the activation signal to the inside of the cell after antigen has been recognized. Whether a particular T cell will interact with antigen presented by a class I or a class II molecule is determined by its CD4 or CD8 accessory molecules. CD4 molecules interact only with MHC class II molecules and CD8 only with class I. Other adhesion molecules stabilize and enhance the interaction between the T cell and the APC (Figure 24).

We might mention here that T cells with γδ receptors are somewhat different. In the first place, they are especially associated with epithelial tissues (skin, gut, etc.) rather than the organized lymphoid tissues. In the second place, they do not appear to necessarily require antigen to be processed and presented to them by APCs. Indeed, they do not seem to interact at all with MHC molecules in the way that T cells with αβ receptors interact.

The parts of the TCR α and β chains that interact with peptide and MHC vary considerably in their amino acid sequence from molecule to molecule, much more than any other parts of the chains. These binding parts are therefore known as the variable (Vα and Vβ) domains, and it is their primary sequence that dictates with which combinations of peptide and MHC they interact effectively. The great polymorphism of the V domains is created by an ingenious genetic mechanism that is also used, as you will see, for creating diversity in antibodies.

The TCR Repertoire

T cells all start life with an identical collection of small *gene segments* in their *germ line DNA*. As each cell matures in the thymus, it selects at random some of these gene segments and rearranges them to build a whole V gene to code for the variable part of the TCR peptide. The segments are in three groups such that the cell uses one V, one D and one J segment to make a unique VDJ gene that codes for the Vβ domain (Figure 25). There are about 25 different Vβ genes (or alleles), 2 different Dβ genes and 12 different Jβ genes, so there are 600 different VDJβ chain combinations. The same mechanisms of *gene recombination* can produce

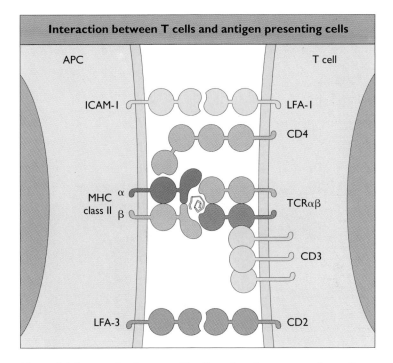

Interaction between T cells and antigen presenting cells

APC   T cell

ICAM-I   LFA-I

CD4

MHC α   TCRαβ
class II β

CD3

LFA-3   CD2

Figure 24. Interaction between T cells and antigen-presenting cells.
This represents some of the molecules that are involved in the direct
interaction between a T cell and an APC. The TCR molecule (composed of an
α and β chain) interacts with peptide presented in an MHC class II (or class I)
molecule on the APC. The CD4 (or CD8) accessory molecule on the T cell
stabilizes the TCR–MHC interaction, so prolonging the contact to allow a signal
to be initiated by the CD3 accessory molecule polypeptides that eventually
activate genes in the T cell nucleus. The adhesion between the cells that is
necessary for the TCR–MHC–peptide interaction to occur in the first place is
made possible by the mutual interaction of adhesion molecules such as ICAM-I,
LFA-I, LFA-3 and CD2 on the T cell and APC.

around 5,000 different α chains, so the random pairing of any
one α and any one β chain will produce more than 360,000 different αβ TCR molecules. In fact the total number, known as the
repertoire, is very much greater than this because there are many
different subtle ways for the VDJ segments to be recombined and
the total potential repertoire of αβ TCR molecules is probably
greater than 10^{17}. Likewise, there are the same sort of number of
different possible γδ TCR combinations. From these calculations
it is obvious that our T cell repertoire contains a potentially enormous number of different specificities, although in practice we
probably use relatively few of them in our life time.   **47**

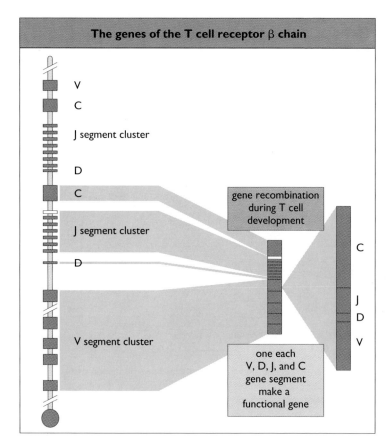

Figure 25. The genes of the T cell receptor β chain.
There are three sets of 'genes' for the TCR polypeptide chains. Gene segments are randomly recombined in individual developing T cells to create functional genes that code for molecules. Illustrated here is just the β set that codes the β chain of the TCR. The arrangements of the genes for the α, γ and δ chains are similar to this, but are on different chromosomes. The way in which the recombination occurs is identical to that used in B cells to code for their immunoglobulin receptors – this is illustrated in Figure 29.

ANTIBODIES

Each antibody molecule consists of one or more basic units each containing four polypeptide chains – two identical heavy (H) chains and two identical light (L) chains – which are assembled in a Y shape. The two arms have the same structure and they are the parts of the molecule that combine with antigen (Figure 26).

When we compare the amino acid sequences in these parts of many different antibody molecules we see that they vary widely.

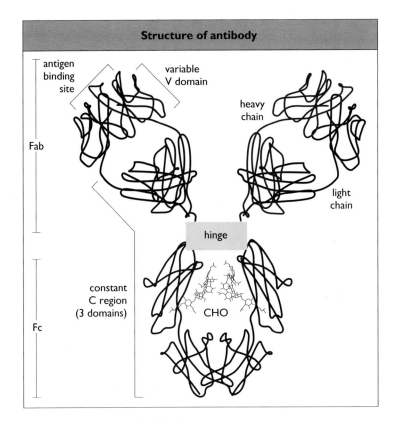

Figure 26. Structure of antibody.
This is a computer simulation of a human IgG molecule showing the two identical light chains (L) and two identical heavy chains (H). In each of the Fab parts of the molecule, the H and L chains each contribute three CDR loops to the binding site for antigen. The Fab parts are joined by a hinge region to the Fc part. The precise structure of the hinge is not known but it allows the Fab parts to move relative to each other, thus making cross-linking of antigens easier to accomplish. In one side of the molecule the H and L chains are shown in different colours. The Fc part of the antibody is concerned with the effector functions of the antibody and is composed of the constant ends of the H chain and some carbohydrate (CHO). Computer-generated image courtesy of Brian Sutton.

As in the TCR molecules, these are called variable (V) regions and it is these that determine the specificity of the antibody. They are the parts of the molecule to which antigen will bind. Thus, different antibodies have different sequences and combine with different antigens. The 'stem' of the molecule is unlike the two arms. It does not combine with antigen and varies much less between different antibodies and it is, in consequence, known as the constant (C) region of the molecule.

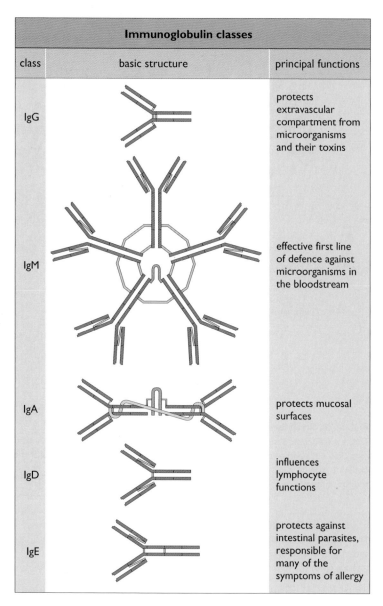

Immunoglobulin classes		
class	basic structure	principal functions
IgG		protects extravascular compartment from microorganisms and their toxins
IgM		effective first line of defence against microorganisms in the bloodstream
IgA		protects mucosal surfaces
IgD		influences lymphocyte functions
IgE		protects against intestinal parasites, responsible for many of the symptoms of allergy

Figure 27. Immunoglobulin classes.
IgG illustrates the basic structure of the immunoglobulin molecule which consists of two identical heavy and two identical light polypeptide chains. IgM is a pentamer of this basic structure, IgA is a dimer (associated with two other protein chains namely the J-chain and the secretory piece) in the form secreted through mucous membranes, IgD differs relatively little from IgG, while IgE possesses an extra globular domain.

There are some differences in the structures of C regions of anti-bodies, however, and these are used to classify them, irrespective of their antigen combining specificity, into immunoglobulin classes which have distinct biological activities manifested when the antibody has combined with its specific antigen. The major classes in man are known as IgG, IgM, IgA, IgD and IgE (Figure 27). The constant parts of the H chain which determine the antibody class are known as μ in IgM, γ in IgG, α in IgA, δ in IgD and ε in IgE. As will be discussed later, each B cell can switch from making one class to another. In all classes, L chains are made of both κ and λ type. Immunologists refer to the third arm of the molecule, which determines the immunoglobulin class and biological function, as the Fc part and to the two arms of the molecule that combine with antigen as the Fab parts.

When antibody molecules are expressed on the surface of B cells, they are synthesized with a small extra domain at the end of the Fc part that anchors the molecule in the cell membrane in

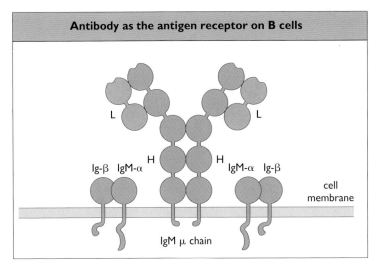

Figure 28. Antibody as the antigen receptor on B cells.
Antibody as the antigen receptor on B cells binds to antigen presented in an undegraded form by specialized APCs in spleen and lymph nodes. The molecules are free to move in the cell membrane of the B cell and it is their aggregation brought about by their interaction with concentrated presented antigen that allows the accessory molecules associated with each immunoglobulin molecule to transmit a signal that activates genes in the nucleus of the B cell. These receptor molecules are identical to the secreted antibodies that the B cell makes except that they have an extra domain on their H chains that anchors the molecules in the cell membrane. IgM is shown here, but immunoglobulins of other classes also act as receptors on B cells.

much the same way as TCR and MHC molecules. Also like the TCR molecule, membrane-bound antibody has some other polypeptide chains associated with it that are important in initiating the activation signal that arises after the antibody has bound antigen (Figure 28). Notice that unlike TCR and MHC molecules, antibodies each have two binding sites for antigen, and they will bind directly to intact proteins without the need for them to be first degraded. Most of the membrane-bound antibody on antigen-reactive B cells is either of the IgM or the IgG class.

The Antibody Repertoire
The diversity of antibody V region structures, and hence the diversity of specificity, is generated by processes like those described earlier for T cells. Each B cell has germ line DNA that contains sets of gene segments which it randomly recombines to produce functioning genes to encode the V regions of the H and the L chains (Figure 29). For the H chain, around 300 V segments, 10 D segments and 4 J segments produce 12,000 V_H combinations. Correspondingly for light chains, around 300 V segments and 4 J segments encode 1,200 V_L combinations. As any H chain can be paired with any particular L chain in an individual B cell during its development, there are at least 14,400,000 antibodies that can be produced in this way! In fact, the number is much larger because of the different ways in which the gene segments can recombine and because of the later effects of *mutation*. Nonetheless, it is impressive that so many antibodies can be produced from less than one thousand gene segments. Until these mechanisms were discovered, scientists were always puzzled that the total DNA of our genome would not be sufficient to accommodate one complete gene for each antibody. Selective recombination of germ line gene segments gets around this problem.

Antibody Synthesis and Class Switching
With the activation of its antibody synthesizing machinery, the B cell produces secretable forms of the molecule (that lack the tail on the Fc region) and these are the antibodies found in the circulation with which you are familiar. There are several interesting events that follow from the activation of B cells. For example, although most begin by secreting IgM antibodies which are characteristic of primary immune responses, many will later switch to making antibodies of one of the other classes: these newer antibodies have exactly the same specificity because they use the original V_H region gene but now in combination with another and different C region gene. This process is known as the *class*

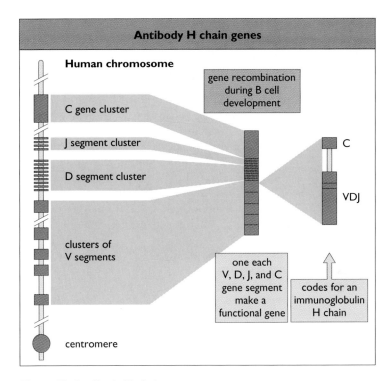

Figure 29. Antibody H chain genes.
The genes that encode the heavy chains of antibody molecules are arranged as shown. As with the TCR genes (Figure 25) there are sets of gene segments, common to all immature B cells, that are randomly recombined to create functional genes to code for H chains. The fact that there are many V, D and J genes to use in this process allows the creation of a very large number of different VDJ combinations, each one of which creates an antibody H chain with a unique amino acid sequence and hence unique specificity for antigen. Although not illustrated, a similar arrangement of gene segments occurs on different chromosomes for the kappa (κ) and lambda (λ) chains, although λ chain variability is much less. The κ and λ gene sets do not, unlike the H sets, contain D segment genes. The mechanism of recombination involves a VDJ recombinase enzyme that recognizes the DNA at just the right points to allow the correct joining at the V–D and D–J junctions. The intervening DNA is no longer available for use, ensuring that an individual cell uses only one set of recombined gene segments to maintain its specificity.

switch for obvious reasons, and leads to production, for example, of IgG antibodies that circulate in the blood and body tissues or IgA antibodies that are secreted across mucous membranes to provide protection in the gut and lungs. The way this is brought about is as follows. The functional gene for an H chain V region is separated from the gene that codes for the constant region of the same polpeptide. By processing the mRNA the V and C genes are brought together to produce a continuous VC peptide. However, as the B cell is stimulated repeatedly by antigen, so it changes the type of H chain it synthesizes, and this process is controlled by various cytokines such as IL-4, IL-5, IL-6, and IFN-γ, produced by CD4$^+$ T cells that drive the class switch. In all cases the cell uses the same recombined VDJ gene as it first used, but reads this in conjunction with another of the C genes that are arranged in sequence on the chromosome, and as the cell switches to making a new immunoglobulin class so the intervening DNA is looped out and not used again. The class switch is related to the generation of memory B cells which may also mutate their VDJ genes thereby causing slight changes in their specificity for antigen.

Mutation of Antibody Genes
Another event that accompanies the growth of B cell clones and the generation of memory B cells is mutation of the genes encoding the V regions of the antibody. This has the effect of slightly changing the amino acid sequences of V regions and hence the fine specificity of the secreted antibody. The major consequence of this is that some of the mutated antibodies bind more strongly, or with a higher *affinity*, to the antigen. This makes them more efficient at bringing about clearance of antigen and its ultimate destruction. So the value of having different classes of antibodies and allowing their affinity to change slightly through mutation is to ensure that the most appropriate and efficient response is made to the particular challenge presented by the antigen. Mutation is another feature of antibodies that makes them different from TCR molecules which, as far as we know, never mutate. The likely explanation for this is that if T cells did mutate they could become autoreactive; remember that most autoreactive T cells are eliminated during their development. Autoreactive B cells on the other hand may be useful physiologically, to promote clearance of dead cells and their debris by phagocytosis, and they do not seem to become involved in autoimmune disease without the help of T cells.

Combination of Antigen and Antibody
The variable Fab regions differ from antibody to antibody in their amino acid sequence and three-dimensional shape. Of course, the sequence determines the shape. One particular antibody molecule will bind to a particular antigen that has a complementary shape. The particular region of the Fab that is involved in this binding is called the combining site and it is

relatively small. The part of the antigen it combines with is also correspondingly small and is called an *antigenic determinant* or epitope. A large antigen molecule, for example the influenza haemagglutinin (one of the coat proteins of the influenza virus) will have many epitopes, each epitope being equivalent in size to a few amino acids. Other antigens, like this, are polyvalent in that they have several different epitopes, or others may have many repeats of the same epitope. Antibodies are divalent (since the basic unit possesses two Fab parts) although IgM and IgA molecules have a higher valency because they are respectively made up from five and two basic divalent units. When antigen and antibody combine, they cross-link to form macromolecular *immune complexes* (Figure 30).

The parts of the antibody molecule most concerned with interaction with antigen are located at the very ends of the Fab parts of the molecule. They are in fact parts of loops of the polypeptide chains that make up the V regions of the H and L chains, which associate in such a way that three loops from each chain come close together to form the binding site. These loops are the areas where the differences in amino acid sequences between different chains are concentrated and are called hyper-variable loops. They determine to which antigen structures the antibody is complementary, so they are also known as *complementarity determining regions* (CDRs). The architecture of the surface made up by the CDR loops permits the molecule to fit closely with antigen epitopes of complementary shape. The strength (affinity) of the ensuing association depends then upon the distribution of various amino acids with particular charges or properties that permit non-covalent bonding to occur between the antibody and the antigen. This is summarized in Figure 31.

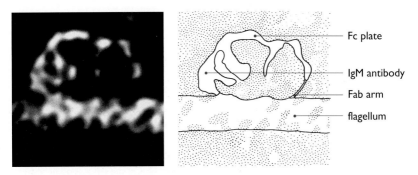

Fc plate

IgM antibody

Fab arm

flagellum

Figure 30. Electron micrograph showing an immune complex.
Shown here is an IgM molecule adopting a crab-like configuration attached to a single flagellum of a bacterium. Courtesy of A Feinstein.

Antibody Idiotypes

Some B cells naturally produce antibodies that react with the parts of the V regions of other antibodies that are involved in binding to antigen. These anti-antibodies are known as anti-idiotype antibodies and the structures they recognize on the other antibody comprise its *idiotype*. Thus, it is possible to identify unique features of antibodies, their idiotypes, by the use of other antibodies. It is largely a matter of convenience which is defined as the idiotype and which as the anti-idiotype. However, as anti-idiotype antibodies may inhibit the idiotype antibody from binding to its antigen you can see that idiotypic interactions with antibody receptors on B cells may be important in regulating lymphocyte activity.

The fact that anti-idiotype antibodies can compete with antigen for the binding site on an antibody (Figure 32) implies that they have some structural similarity to the antigen itself. These are known as *internal images* of external antigens. It is possible to immunize an experimental animal with an anti-idiotype

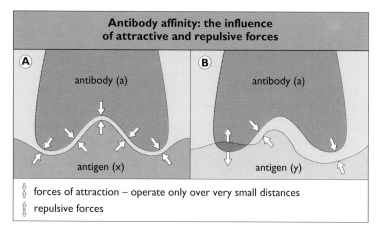

Figure 31. Antibody affinity: the influence of attractive and repulsive forces.
The ability of antibody and antigen to bind together depends initially upon how closely their shapes are complementary. Shape in this sense is determined by the electron clouds that define the surfaces of the molecules. If they do come close together, then the distribution of interacting charged groups on their surfaces will determine how tightly they bind to each other. We refer to the strength of this binding as the affinity of the interaction: high affinity antibodies bind to antigen better than low affinity antibodies. On the left a good fit and high affinity interaction is shown; on the right the same antibody does not fit well or interact strongly with a slightly different antigen and this is an example of low affinity interaction.

antibody and induce the production of more antibody of the same specificity as the antibody bearing the original idiotype. So, antibody responses do not necessarily need antigen to stimulate them. This offers an exciting prospect of using anti-idiotype antibodies as vaccines, and they could be especially useful where the antigen is either toxic or very hard to purify. Several anti-idiotype vaccines are in development as surrogates for vaccines against viruses, for example, hepatitis B virus.

The complementary nature of the idiotype–anti-idiotype pairs also has other interesting implications. For example, anti-idiotype antibodies against anti-hormone (e.g. insulin) antibodies may be able to bind to the specific receptor for the hormone, and thereby mimic the action of the original hormone.

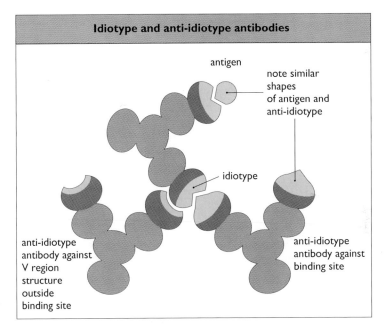

Idiotype and anti-idiotype antibodies

antigen

note similar shapes of antigen and anti-idiotype

idiotype

anti-idiotype antibody against V region structure outside binding site

anti-idiotype antibody against binding site

Figure 32. Idiotype and anti-idiotype antibodies.
The repertoire of antibodies made by one individual is very large and diverse in antigen binding specificity. Amongst the antibodies it is common that some interact with each other through their antigen-binding V regions. These are idiotypic interactions: each antibody expresses its own idiotype and others that react with it are called anti-idiotype antibodies. These may bind to determinants close to the antigen-binding site or with the binding site itself. Anti-idiotype antibodies are made naturally in the course of immune responses and are probably important in regulating responses. Those against the binding site itself may have an overall shape similar to the antigen to which the antibody binds.

57

Antibody Effector Functions

The combination of antibody with antigen is a physico-chemical reaction involving non-covalent bonding, in many respects analogous to the combination of enzyme with its substrate. Antibodies, however, do not directly damage antigens, but rather the combination of the two leads to a variety of different biological events (Figure 33). Although antibodies may alone directly

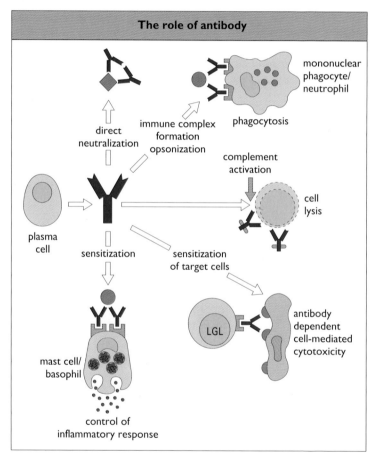

Figure 33. The role of antibody.
The variable parts of the antibody bind to antigen, and once this complex has been formed, then the effector functions are brought into play. They depend upon sites in the constant or Fc part of the molecule that bind either to various Fc receptors or to components of the complement system. Different classes of antibodies are characterized by their individual heavy chains that have unique Fc structures. Accordingly, antibodies of different classes are dedicated to different functions after they have bound antigen.

neutralize toxins produced by bacteria, the destruction or removal of an antigen requires the involvement of other molecules and cells of the immune system. It is the Fc parts of antibodies that determine this involvement in secondary interactions. This nicely illustrates that different parts or domains of antibodies are dedicated to different functions: the V regions bind antigens with immunological specificity; the C regions combine with other molecules and cells (without demonstrating any immunological specificity in the process) to achieve the removal and destruction of the antigen.

Fc Receptors

One major activity of antibodies is to bind to receptors for their Fc regions (FcR) that are expressed on various cells. Some of these are listed in Table 5. You will see that some FcRs tend to

Fc receptors for immunoglobulins		
Receptor	Location	Function
FcγRI	Macrophages	Binds IgG immune complexes, ADCC
FcγRII	Macrophages, polymorphs	Binds free antibodies, phagocytosis, ADCC
FcγRIIIA	NK cells, macrophages, kidney, placenta	Transport of antibodies, ADCC
FcγRIIIB	Neutrophils	Binds IgG immune complexes, stimulates respiratory burst
FcεRI	Mast cells, basophils	Binds IgE, releases inflammatory mediators
FcεRII (various forms)	Inflammatory cells	Regulates B cells, binds IgE for ADCC of parasites
FcαR	Macrophages, polymorphs, T cells, B cells, NK cells	Phagocytosis of IgA immune complexes, ADCC
FcμR	Macrophages, B cells, T cells	Phagocytosis of IgM immune complexes, regulates lymphocyte activity

Table 5. Fc receptors for immunoglobulins.
Receptors for immunoglobulin Fc structures exist on a wide range of immune effector cells. Distribution of receptors ensures that different cells depend upon different classes of immunoglobulins for the expression of their activities. Not all IgG subclasses bind equally well to the Fc receptors. Only FcγRII and FcεRI have affinities high enough to bind respectively IgG and IgE antibodies not yet complexed to antigen.

bind antibody of particular classes (antibodies of different classes have different H chains and hence different Fc structures), and in some cases do so only after the antibody has combined with antigen. Binding of antibodies to Fc receptors is an integral part of the process of phagocytosis and extracellular killing (ADCC) by macrophages, eosinophils and K cells. It is also central to the activation of mast cells and basophils, it has a role in platelet function, and is important in the transport of immunoglobulins of particular classes across the placenta (IgG) and the mucosal surfaces (IgA).

MONOCLONAL ANTIBODIES

As you have seen, individual B cells each make their own particular antibody, but in response to immunization with even a simple antigen, many different B cells will be activated. There are many situations, however, where it would be very valuable to have just one antibody of defined specificity in large amounts. Through the artificial process of cell cloning this is possible. The two important principles involved in this are applied to B cells from an immunized human or animal (Figure 34). First, immune lymphocytes are hybridized with immortal myeloma (a B cell tumour) cells by a process of cell fusion. The hybrid cells so produced have the two valuable properties of both making specific antibody, a trait inherited from the immune B cells, and being immortal in tissue culture, a trait inherited from the tumour cell. The second crucial step is the physical separation (cloning) of hybrid cells from each other, so that individual cells can be persuaded to grow as continuous cloned cell lines *in vitro*. Each clone makes its own antibody hence the term *monoclonal antibody*.

This process was first successfully described by Cesar Milstein and Georges Köhler using rodent lymphocytes – this discovery led to them being awarded the Nobel prize – but it is applicable to other species too. This technology completely revolutionized the way antibodies are made and used. Monoclonal antibodies are extensively used in *immunoassays* for thousands of different compounds and materials and have many applications in preparative procedures and, very importantly, in various types of therapy for human and animal disease. Because the cloned *hybridoma* cells are immortal and grow continuously they can be distributed throughout the world to provide standardized antibodies to everyone who needs them. They also considerably reduce the need to use animals for repeated immunization programmes to produce antisera.

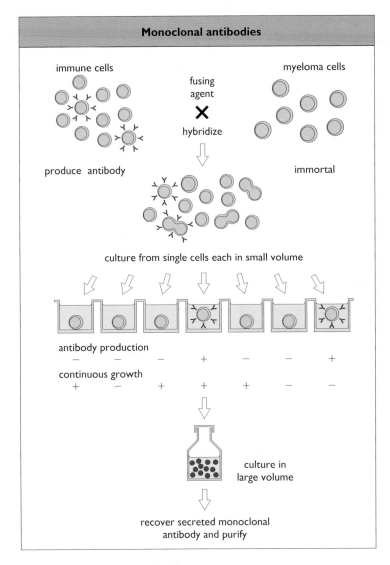

Figure 34. Monoclonal antibodies.
Lymphocytes from an immunized mouse, rat or human, are mixed with myeloma cells and exposed to a fusing agent such as polyethylene glycol. If the conditions are carefully controlled, some cells hybridize and some of these both make specific antibody and will survive indefinitely in culture. These are separated from the other cells by growing them individually and then using the clone to establish permanent large cultures from which the monoclonal antibodies can be harvested. Typically, a few different monoclonal antibodies can be recovered from a hundred million lymphocytes, so this is not a method that recovers all the antibody-forming cells.

61

Engineering the Antibody Molecule

Recent advances have opened up new possibilities for using antibodies. They relate to engineering the antibody molecule by inserting and changing specific parts such as V or Fc regions to customize its function as illustrated in Figure 35. The 1987

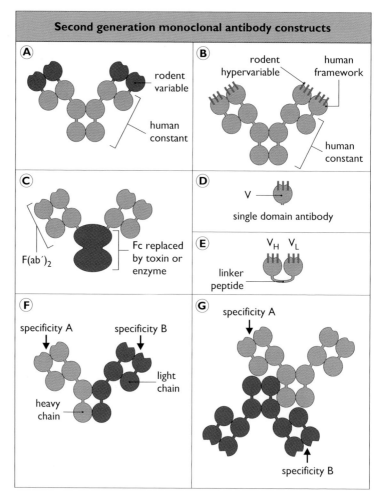

Figure 35. Genetically engineered antibodies.
Through manipulating the gene segments that code for antibody L and H chains, it is possible to construct molecules of various forms. (A) Chimaeric antibody. (B) Humanized reshaped antibody with specificity of original rodent antibody. (C) Antibody–toxin/enzyme chimaeric molecule. (D) Single V domain peptide. (E) Single chain Fv molecule made from linked V domains from an H and an L chain. (F and G) Bi-specific antibodies made by protein engineering.

Nobel Prize winner Susumu Tonegawa recognized that discrete gene fragments coded separately for the variable and constant parts of the immunoglobulin molecules. Genetic engineers then cloned antibodies with improved or novel properties by isolating the DNA coding for the variable part of one antibody, and combining it with the genes coding for the constant domains of an unrelated immunoglobulin. Because it is easier to manipulate the immune system of the rat by selective immunization, a number of rodent monoclonal antibodies have been made that have potential clinical benefit. The disadvantage is that rat immunoglobulin evokes an immune response in the human because it is a foreign protein. One way round this problem is to link the genes coding for the variable portion of rodent antibodies to those coding for the constant region of human immunoglobulin.

The *chimaeric antibodies* made from these recombinant genes have distinct therapeutic advantages. In the first place, because they are predominantly human they are less likely to evoke an immune response and therefore safer to inject into patients than whole rodent antibodies. Secondly, we can select constant region genes which will give the antibody those effector functions which are suited to a particular application. For example, lytic antibodies are preferable in some therapeutic situations, so the most appropriate choice is to use genes coding for the constant regions of the complement-fixing human IgG1 or IgG3 subclasses. Conversely, antibodies to be used for imaging (localizing) tumours, cardiac infarcts or blood clots benefit from the constant region of the weakly cytophilic IgG4 subclass that binds poorly to the Fc receptors which exist on many cells, and which does not activate the complement system.

There are more precise ways in which useful antibody specificities can be created. Because antibodies have much the same structure in different species, one can take very small parts of the structure of the antibody and insert it into another. By knowing the gene sequence of a useful rodent antibody, just those parts that code for the hypervariable loops that determine binding specificity can be used to replace the analogous parts of a human antibody. This is the process of making reshaped or humanized antibodies. The resultant recombinant gene codes for an antibody which displays the specificity of the original rodent antibody even though it is otherwise human in structure and nature. This process has been applied to antibodies used in the management of malignant and infectious diseases, transplant rejection and autoimmune reactions. In this regard it is interesting to note that humanized antibodies have been used successfully to treat a

63

ACQUIRED IMMUNITY

tumour of white blood cells (a lymphoma) and severe rheumatoid arthritis. Furthermore, humanized antibodies to herpes
simplex virus, respiratory syncytial virus, HIV and bacterial toxins
have been developed and are currently being used or tested for
use clinically. Antibodies of the last kind are especially valuable
in the treatment of shock resulting from infection with Gram-
negative bacteria.

We have emphasized at several points how the specificity of an
antibody depends on the precise sequence of amino acids in the
hypervariable loops. Even small changes in these can affect its
specificity and this is actually what happens when antibody genes
mutate naturally in the course of an immune response. Some of
these mutations increase the affinity of the antibody for antigen,
which is very important to its biological effectiveness. Starting
with a cloned antibody, it is possible to reproduce this process
artificially through *site-directed mutagenesis* (Figure 36) to change
V gene sequences to produce antibodies of higher affinity, valuable in therapy, or antibodies of lower affinity that might be pre-
pared for imaging or antibody-based preparative procedures.

Repertoire Cloning

Antibody engineering techniques have depended until recently
on the initial availability of relatively large amounts of genetic
material and hence an abundant supply of cells making specific
antibody. However, the polymerase chain reaction (PCR)
method makes many copies of one gene, and so enables us to
isolate and express the antibody genes from even a single cell.
This same technique, coupled with developments in antibody
detection and expression has also been used to isolate libraries
of antibody genes from mixtures of lymphoid cells that are
making antibodies with a wide range of specificities. This powerful procedure, which is known as repertoire cloning and is illustrated in Figure 37, provides a way both to the rapid production
of a new range of monoclonal antibodies and to the analysis of
the antibody repertoire in normal and other individuals. Its value
in circumventing some of the problems that limit the development and application of conventional human monoclonal antibodies is being explored. These include the limited supply of
specifically immune lymphocytes and the instability and low antibody secreting capacity of immortalized human hybrid cell lines.

THE COMPLEMENT SYSTEM

Immune complexes of antigen and antibody are frequently
ingested by phagocytic cells and destroyed intracellularly. This
appears to be the fate of most foreign materials against which

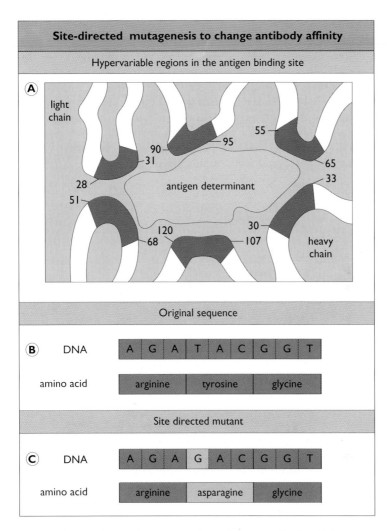

Site-directed mutagenesis to change antibody affinity

Hypervariable regions in the antigen binding site

(A) light chain

55
90
95
31
65
33
28
antigen determinant
51
30
120
107
68
heavy chain

Original sequence

(B) DNA | A | G | A | T | A | C | G | G | T |

amino acid | arginine | tyrosine | glycine |

Site directed mutant

(C) DNA | A | G | A | G | A | C | G | G | T |

amino acid | arginine | asparagine | glycine |

Figure 36. Site-directed mutagenesis to change antibody affinity.
(A) The six hypervariable CDR loops of an antibody contribute to binding the antigen. (B) Knowing the gene sequence of the CDR loops allows a new nucleotide sequence to be created by targetting the gene with a primer of the new sequence. (C) The mutated gene has a new sequence and codes for a different peptide sequence, thus affecting the strength of the antigen binding (affinity).

antibodies are produced. However, the fate of immune complexes also depends very heavily upon their ability to activate the complement system. This system consists of more than twenty components which act in a cascade to bring about destruction of

microorganisms, stimulation of inflammatory reactions and pro-
motion of the phagocytosis of immune complexes (Figure 38).

Some activities of the complement system depend upon the
presence of complement receptors (CRs) for particular complement components on different cell types. For example, phagocytosis is enhanced by the C3b component and there are receptors
for this on phagocytic cells. From this it can be seen that phagocytosis involving antibody and complement (see Figure 14) will
depend for its efficiency upon the expression of both Fc receptors and C3b receptors on the phagocytic cells.

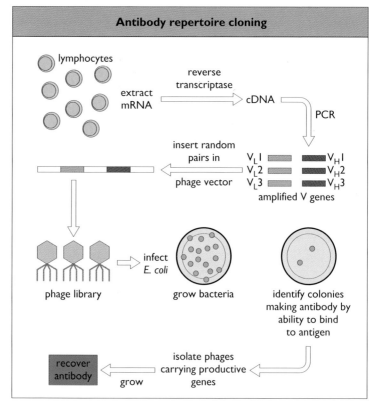

Figure 37. Antibody repertoire cloning.
Similar in principle to making monoclonal antibodies (Figure 35) but here
antibody fragments are isolated and cloned in phages that grow in the bacteria
Escherichia coli. Very large numbers of different antibody specificities can be
recovered by this method because PCR methods initially make many copies of
individual V genes and also the growth and cloning efficiency is much greater
than that of lymphocytes in conventional hybridoma technology.

Opsonization, Lysis and Inflammation

The process of opsonization is illustrated in Figure 38, together with the other main physiological functions of complement. The interaction of antibody (through its Fc region) with complement

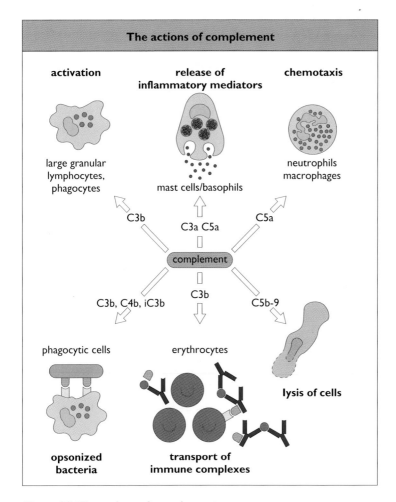

The actions of complement

activation

release of inflammatory mediators

chemotaxis

large granular lymphocytes, phagocytes

mast cells/basophils

neutrophils macrophages

C3b

C3a C5a

C5a

complement

C3b, C4b, iC3b

C3b

C5b-9

phagocytic cells

erythrocytes

lysis of cells

opsonized bacteria

transport of immune complexes

Figure 38. The actions of complement.
This is a system of more than twenty proteins that circulate in the blood and body tissues. Some are enzymes that work in a cascade: one becomes active, cleaves another to activate it, and so on. At the centre is component C3 which can be activated by, for example, antibodies aggregated in immune complexes or by some bacterial compounds that first bind and activate other complement proteins that cleave C3 to activate it. The C3b and C3a degradation products have direct opsonizing, chemotactic and inflammatory effects and also activate the so-called lytic pathway involving C5 to C9.

does not necessarily lead directly to phagocytosis; it may also lead to the lysis of cells to which the antibodies have bound. Complement-dependent lysis of this type is important in destroying certain bacteria and also in blood transfusion reactions. According to the size of immune complexes of antibody and antigen, complement may be involved in facilitating their transport from the blood to the liver and spleen where they are then phagocytosed by the resident macrophages. Type 1 complement receptors (CR1) on red blood cells bind immune complexes and the red cells carry them to the macrophages in the liver. If the receptors are not present in their usual physiological amounts, then complexes may persist and cause inflammation in various tissues, as in some rheumatic diseases.

Complement promotes local inflammation mainly through generating chemotactic stimuli for neutrophils and monocytes/macrophages and through producing components that degranulate mast cells and basophils.

Control of Complement Activation
The complement system has an enormous potential to cause inflammation, and so there are several important control mechanisms that limit its activity. They include, for example, ways to stop the breakdown of C3 further catalyzing its own breakdown and factors that promote decay of activated C3. Such is the importance of complement to the proper functioning of the immune system that genetic deficiencies of particular complement components may lead to severe diseases, such as chronic infections and immune complex diseases. In the latter, complexes of antigen and antibody are not effectively cleared by phagocytic cells and they become lodged in the tissues where they initiate local inflammation. We will consider examples of these in a later section.

IMMUNE RESPONSES

The cells and molecules that interact together to provide natural non-specific immunity are obviously very effective at preventing infection. We must remember that our body is continuously exposed to microorganisms but it rarely suffers ill effects from them. However, as a result of the evolutionary contest between parasites and their hosts there are many ways in which microorganisms can avoid destruction after they infect a host and, in doing so, cause disease. The immune system, and particularly the adaptive immune system, is always available and ready to deal with infection. It is designed to protect the host against the five classes of infectious organisms, namely viruses, bacteria, fungi, protozoa and helminths. Infectious diseases, with parasites in particular, present enormous problems worldwide with hundreds of millions of people being affected. Recently, new problems have emerged associated with infections such as HIV and the Legionnaires' disease bacterium, the evolution of drug-resistant malarial parasites, increased hospital infection with antibiotic-resistant bacteria and the 'opportunistic' infections in the increased numbers of patients who are immunosuppressed by drugs. In addition, the very modern phenomenon of large scale international travel greatly helps the spread of infectious diseases.

When discussing infectious disease we have to distinguish between the infection itself and the associated disease. Infection refers simply to the presence in the body of the microorganism. If the agent persists in the body but causes no damage then the person is called a carrier and the infection is sub-clinical. Infections cannot be identified easily until it has become sufficiently active to cause disease. A carrier is potentially dangerous if the organism that persists is excreted, as in typhoid disease, for example. Disease will only be obvious either if the microorganism itself damages or kills cells of the host or if the body's immune response to the infection also damages host tissue in its efforts to destroy the parasite.

In the sections that follow we will describe the different types of adaptive responses that are important in providing resistance to infections by different groups of microorganisms. **69**

Subsequently, those responses which cause damage to the body when expressed in an extreme or exaggerated way will be described. As you have seen in the first part of this book, adaptive immune responses are highly complex in terms of the interactions of cells and molecules involved in them, and the magnitude of the adaptive immune response usually increases specifically on subsequent encounter with antigen. However, we should note that the immune system functions less effectively in elderly people. This suggests that we may have a limited store of potentially useful lymphocytes and that this can become exhausted through use; the natural mechanisms of immunity also probably become less effective with increasing age. It is likely that changes in the patterns of cytokine production underlie these changes.

IMMUNITY TO BACTERIA

The nature of the immune response to bacteria varies according to whether the organisms grow extracellularly or intracellularly. If extracellular, immune responses tend to be rapidly effective and involve antibody. However, if the bacteria divide intracellularly, they may survive for a long time, and immune responses are not always very effective and tend to involve T cells. Toxins secreted by bacteria can usually be neutralized by antibodies: it is obvious that rapid immune responses are necessary to avoid damage by toxins such as those produced by *Clostridium welchii* which causes gas gangrene.

Anti-bacterial Killing Mechanisms
When studying the ways in which immune mechanisms cause the destruction of bacteria and the ways in which bacteria in turn avoid this destruction, you will see in some but not all cases, examples of the dynamic interplay between the immune system and the parasite. For example, not all toxins are equally well neutralized by antibodies, some actually poison phagocytes. Further, bacteria that normally replicate inside phagocytes may be helped by antibody to enter the cells in which they favour living. Mycobacteria are an example of this, they are very difficult to destroy and can live for many years inside macrophages.

In other cases, if the bacteria have a capsule or adhere only poorly to phagocytic cells, they are better able to resist being killed. For example, ten meningococci (bacteria with a capsule) can kill a mouse, whereas if the capsule is removed by enzymes more than ten thousand are needed because the organisms are so much more susceptible to phagocytosis and intracellular killing. The staphylococci are examples of bacteria that defend themselves against immune attack by another evasion mechanism. They produce endotoxins that damage neutrophils and prevent their chemotaxis to sites of infection.

Opsonization. We have stressed earlier how important phagocytosis is in protective immunity and in the case of many bacteria this is the main route of their destruction. As was seen in Figure 14, the presence of antibody greatly increases the rate of clearance of bacteria from the blood by phagocytosis. When complement is also present, the clearance is even faster. Some organisms are also killed directly by complement-dependent lysis, the activation of the lytic process being initiated by antibody binding to the surface of the bacteria.

Similarly, complement components that have been fixed on the bacterial cell wall also bind to complement receptors on a variety of cells thereby enhancing their removal. The importance of the complement system can also be seen in those individuals who inherit deficiencies in their complement system. Some of them suffer persistent bacterial infections which may be fatal.

However, antibodies made specifically in response to infection are very important, not only in aiding the phagocytosis of bacteria, but also in coating the bacteria to make them susceptible to attack by cytotoxic cells. The major roles of antibody in bacterial infection have been summarized in Figure 33. Not all bacteria are equally susceptible to the effects of complement. Some, for example, have cell walls very resistant to lysis, and others interfere with the complement activation processes or increase the rate of breakdown of complement components.

Secretory Immune System

Many bacteria, and the same is true of viruses, are encountered at mucous membranes. Apart from the natural immune mechanisms associated with these membranes, which we discussed earlier, they are also specially equipped with IgA type antibodies. These can bind to microorganisms and prevent their adherence to the cells of the mucous membrane thereby preventing infection and stopping the replication of the bacteria. IgA antibodies are also made against toxins secreted by some bacteria and they similarly prevent them entering the body.

IgA gives such protection in tears, saliva, bronchial secretions and in the gut. If mucous barriers are breached, IgE antibodies bound to mast cells provide the next line of defence. When triggered by the infectious agent, histamine and other chemicals are

71

released which enhance the local immune response by increasing the passage of cells, antibody and complement from the circulation to the infected site (Figure 39). This illustrates the protective value of inflammatory responses.

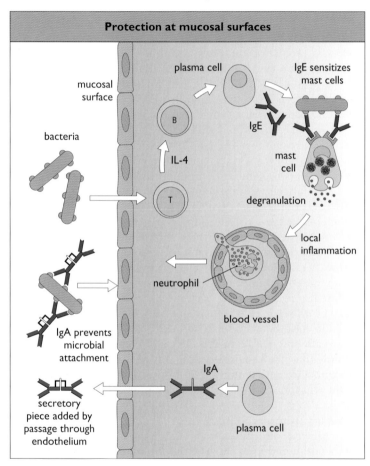

Figure 39. Protection at mucosal surfaces.
About half of our lymphocytes are associated with mucosal tissues of the gut, lungs, etc. Although mucosal lymphocytes can circulate to other parts of the body, their special function is to make antibodies of the IgA and IgE types, with the help of mucosal-associated T cells that make IL-4. Between them, these antibodies either prevent the attachment of microbes to the mucosal epithelial cells (IgA), or if antigens penetrate into mucosal tissues, then provide the stimuli through mast cell and basophil degranulation for local inflammation (IgE) – imagine this as a response designed to prevent antigen spreading to the rest of the body. IgE-mediated immunity is important in resistance to some parasites and also in allergies such as hay fever and asthma.

The Role of T Cells in Immunity to Bacteria

Some bacteria, for example the TB organism, *Mycobacterium tuberculosis*, can survive and divide inside macrophages after being phagocytosed. It escapes being killed in the cell by resisting the attack of enzymes and reactive oxygen intermediates, and also by inhibiting the fusion of the lysosome with the phagosome in the macrophage. The only way in which macrophages eventually kill mycobacteria depends upon them becoming activated by the action of cytokines made by $CD4^+$ T cells. In addition, because infected macrophages express mycobacterial antigens on their surface, they may also be susceptible to the cytolytic attack of T cells.

However, it is obvious that many people encounter this particular infectious agent and become immune to it, as demonstrated by their resistance to infection (or reinfection) and by their positive delayed skin test to an antigenic extract (tuberculin) of the organism. Such tests are used widely to identify people who are immune to infection by particular organisms. The key to the immune protection is T cell activation. In animals, immunity to TB can be transferred from one individual to another with T cells, but not with B cells or antibody. T cell deficiencies that are inherited or acquired (e.g. AIDS), render an individual animal or human more susceptible to infection caused by microorganisms such as TB, as well as other organisms, such as fungi, which can grow intracellularly.

The activation of T cells by antigen leads to the production of a variety of soluble products, mediators of inflammation including cytokines. Perhaps only one T cell in 10,000 or even 100,000 recognizes the infectious agent. This would hardly seem to be adequate to keep us free from infection but there is a considerable local amplification due to cytokines which promote cell division, activate macrophages (especially important with TB) and attract other cells (*chemotaxis*) non-specifically. $CD4^+$ T cells may also have a role as cytotoxic cells – a function we usually associate with $CD8^+$ T cells – in this sort of infection. In spite of all these immune mechanisms, TB organisms may still survive and grow inside the inflammatory granulomas that form around them, causing the gross destruction seen in Figure 40.

It might be imagined therefore that if one specific immune response is initiated, for example to *M. tuberculosis*, the various amplification factors may also provide (non-specific) protection against another organism that lives intracellularly, for example *Listeria*, present at the same time but to which specific immunity is lacking. This is exactly the case.

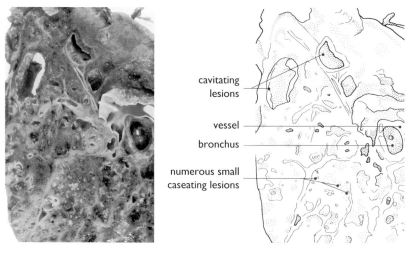

cavitating
lesions

vessel

bronchus

numerous small
caseating lesions

Figure 40. Tuberculosis.
This lung shows damage due to infection with *Mycobacterium tuberculosis*. The
bacteria continues to grow inside cells causing the immune response to
produce fibrosis and granuloma formation. This can lead to caseation causing
further lung damage. Fibrosed lungs were a very common occurrence before
antibiotic treatment of TB. Courtesy of Professor Neville Woolf.

IMMUNITY TO VIRAL INFECTION

Viruses have an absolute dependency upon the cells of the body.
Because they can only replicate intracellularly, special forms of
immune reaction are needed to eliminate them. Macrophages
readily take up viruses in a non-specific way and kill them.
However, if the virus does multiply intracellularly, the cell may
be killed, as may the host. This illustrates the direct tissue-damaging effects (pathology) that some viruses have. Antibodies
cannot normally penetrate cells and can only provide protection
when the virus is outside cells. So, we need two kinds of immune
reaction to the virus; first an antibody response which affects the
virus outside cells and in the circulation, and secondly, a true
cell-mediated response to reach the intracellular virus. These
important responses are summarized in Figure 41, but before
describing the immune mechanisms that deal with virus infection, it is worth considering the peculiar nature of the influenza
virus that ensures we suffer repeatedly from influenza. This illustrates why it can be so difficult to establish effective immunity in
the population against some viruses.

Shift and Drift of Influenza Virus Antigens

A flu vaccine that seems to work this year, probably against last year's strain of virus, may not work next year. This is because the surface coat of the virus changes and an immune response to last year's antigen is not specific for this year's antigen.

Influenza virus, like many others, undergoes shift and drift. The virus attaches to cells by its haemagglutinin molecules; these

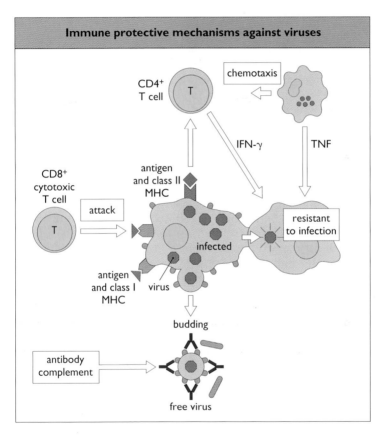

Figure 41. Immune protective mechanisms against viruses.
Viruses have an absolute need to infect a cell and replicate inside it. In most cases, cells infected with virus have viral antigen that associates with MHC class I molecules on their surface, which is recognized by CD8$^+$ T cells which lyse the infected cell. Also, CD4$^+$ T cells recognize viral antigen associated with MHC class II molecules and these cells, and macrophages, release cytokines that act on other nearby tissue cells to make them resistant to further infection by virus. If free virus is secreted by infected cells, it may be bound by anti-viral antibodies that, through the activation of complement, may lead to lysis of viral particles or promote their phagocytosis.

are antigens, and if they change only a little (antigenic drift) there is still enough similarity in the shape of their epitopes to be recognized by the immune memory cells generated by a previous response to the original virus. However, if there has been a major change (antigenic shift), then the protective immunity is lost. The common cold virus (rhinovirus) uses a similar technique to evade protective immunity, which is why immunization for this very common infection does not work.

Role of Antibody in Protection Against Viruses
It is quite likely that IgA antibody secreted locally in the nose and lung may be helpful in protection against many virus infections. However, its effectiveness is limited by antigenic shift in the antigens of the virus. Antibodies of the IgM or IgG types are also generally made in response to virus infection and these circulate in the blood and tissue fluids to provide protection throughout the body. Antibody can neutralize virus by blocking its entry into cells, thereby preventing virus multiplication, and it can also destroy free virus particles by activating complement.

Interestingly, the further the virus has to travel from its port of entry into the body to the tissue which it finally affects, the more effective is antibody-based protection. A good example of this is poliomyelitis where the virus has to travel from the gut to the brain. However, because viruses in general can very rapidly invade cells and replicate, a primary antibody response often cannot be made quickly enough to combat the first infection with a particular virus. Thus, you can see that specific antibody is much more effective in dealing with a virus the second, rather than the first time it infects the host. However, in both situations, immunity provided by T cells is crucially important in eradicating infection once the virus is located inside the cells.

Reactions of T Cells Against Viruses Inside Cells
Cells infected with many types of virus express viral antigens on their surface membranes. These can be recognized by CD8$^+$ T-cytotoxic cells which destroy the virus-infected cell. The destruction of tissues is the price we pay for destroying the place in which virus is replicating. Incomplete virus particles released from lysed cells are not infective and complete virus particles are exposed to, and neutralized by, antibodies and complement.

The value of T cell immunity against virus infection is shown in those children who, because of a T cell deficiency, cannot cope with virus infections, contrasted with those who are are immunoglobulin deficient who can. This simplification is not true of all virus infections but is true of a group of viruses which include herpes (shingles and glandular fever), smallpox and rubella. One of the triumphs of medicine has been the eradication of smallpox through the universal use of an effective vaccine. A key factor that has contributed to this success is the fact that the smallpox virus shows very little drift so that one vaccine was effective for everyone.

CD4$^+$ T-helper cells will also recognize viral antigen on the surface of infected cells. These T cells release chemotactic factors and cytokines, including IFN-γ and TNF, that activate cells in such a way that they become resistant to viral infection. When somebody has recovered from a natural virus infection they have T cells that are cytotoxic to virally-infected cells, specific antibody against the virus and long-lived immunity.

HUMAN IMMUNODEFICIENCY VIRUS (HIV) AND ACQUIRED IMMUNODEFICIENCY SYNDROME (AIDS)

HIV has some very distinctive properties that make it difficult for the immune system to control this infection and make it impossible for the virus to be eliminated once it has infected the body. The virus is illustrated in Figure 42. You can best understand these difficult properties by examining how the virus infects people and how the illness it causes develops (Figure 43).

HIV is a sexually transmitted virus which is passed by heterosexual or homosexual intercourse from one partner to the other. It is transmitted either as free virus or as infected cells. In some people, not all, there is an early illness involving fever, skin rash etc, which is like the effects of many other virus infections and may be quite unremarkable. This then resolves and a period without obvious clinical symptoms, the asymptomatic phase, follows which can last for many years. What happens immediately after infection is that the RNA in the virus is copied as DNA and becomes integrated into the DNA of the infected cell. The early viral illness is a result of viral replication at this time: viral protein antigen is shed and may be detected in the circulation. This is followed by an antibody response and the detection of either antigen or antibody is evidence of HIV infection.

While the antibody response continues (there is also an accompanying response of anti-viral T cells), the disease is quiescent in the asymptomatic phase largely because the virus does not replicate. Because its genetic material persists, however, the infection as such is not cleared by the immune response. Gradually, the levels of T cells fall although the loss of CD4$^+$ T cells is greater than CD8$^+$ cells; hence clinicians measure the CD4$^+$:CD8$^+$ T cell ratio in the blood to monitor progress of the disease.

77

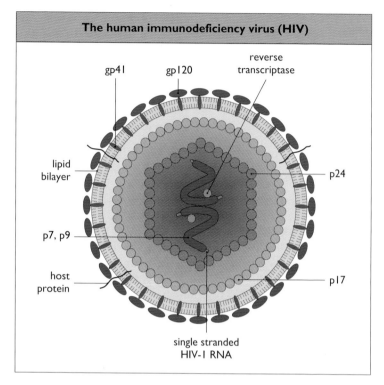

The human immunodeficiency virus (HIV)

gp41 gp120 reverse transcriptase

lipid bilayer

p24

p7, p9

host protein

p17

single stranded HIV-1 RNA

Figure 42. The human immunodeficiency virus.
HIV is the virus that causes AIDS. The genetic material, RNA, is packaged in the centre in various core proteins (p7, p9, p17, p24). The outside is covered in the array of envelope coat proteins, one of which (gp120) is responsible for binding to the CD4 molecules on cell surfaces that the virus uses as its means of entering the cell. Once inside, a DNA copy of the RNA is made using the reverse transcriptase enzyme and is inserted into the genes of the host cell. This becomes an integrated viral genome and can remain quiet for many years, but when it becomes activated it begins to produce the various proteins and RNA to assemble whole infective virus particles.

Infections and Tumours

The disease of AIDS appears when the levels of $CD4^+$ T cells reach catastrophically low levels. At this time, because the host's effective immunity is so compromised or deficient, strange and unusual opportunistic infections appear as well as tumours, such as Kaposi's sarcoma. It is a combination of infection and malignancy that is the cause of death. We basically do not know what are the stimuli for the appearance of the full AIDS disease which in some people is preceded by a phase known as the AIDS-related complex (ARC). However, it is thought that stimuli that

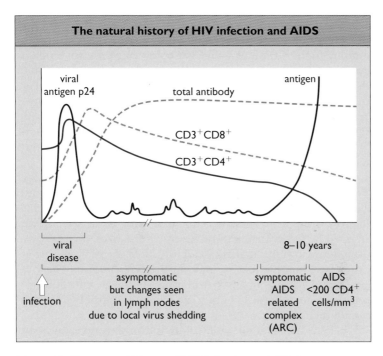

Figure 43. The natural history of HIV infection and AIDS.
There are four distinct phases associated with HIV infection. In many, but not all
people, the first is a brief, mild viral disease that immediately follows the
infection. At this stage, the viral p24 antigen can be found in the circulation. The
second is a long asymptomatic phase, when as the name implies, there are no
obvious outward signs of disease. However, during this phase there are changes
to the distribution of cells in the lymphoid tissues, and in the blood the numbers
of T cells begin to decline, with relatively more CD4$^+$ than CD8$^+$ cells
disappearing. Evidence of infection can be seen through the presence in the
blood of antibodies (some of which, e.g. anti-envelope, remain high throughout
infection) and anti-viral cytotoxic CD8$^+$ T cells. When the numbers of
circulating T cells become very low, but with CD8$^+$ cells outnumbering CD4$^+$
cells, then the third stage can be seen; this may be very brief and is known as the
AIDS-related complex (ARC) phase in which gross changes in lymph nodes take
place and viral antigen is again found in the circulation. The prelude to this stage
is the activation of the dormant integrated viral genes in infected cells. The final
stage, AIDS proper, which may not appear until many years after the initial
infection, is when catastrophically low levels of T cells are reached, so
compromising the immune system that tumours and many otherwise rare
infections become commonplace and are fatal.

activate the infected cells, in turn activating the dormant viral
genes, may be responsible.

Why the T cells die is something of a mystery too. We know that the virus infects T-helper cells and macrophages through binding to the CD4 molecules that both cell types express via its gp120 surface protein. As these cells are distributed throughout the body, there are many sites that become infected. It appears that T cells can be killed in a variety of ways: by the activity of anti-viral $CD8^+$ T cells; by autoantibodies formed for some reason against the cells themselves; by direct lysis by the virus; or by programmed cell death (*apoptosis*) induced by unknown means.

Treatment

The treatment of AIDS therefore presents one of the great challenges to medical science. The search for a vaccine is constrained by the strange natural history of the virus, but there are no reasons to think that the search is futile. At present, various drugs have some effect in limiting the replication of the viral genes, and these coupled with the prevention of infection by a healthy general life-style help some patients control the progression of their disease.

There is considerable confusion and misinformation about this disease. Although it is clearly transmitted sexually, HIV can also be passed from infected mothers to their babies, either in the womb, or as suckling infants, but this does not happen in every case. HIV is also a potential contaminant of blood and blood products, so there are many cases of recipients of blood transfusions becoming infected and haemophiliacs who have become infected through using contaminated factor VIII, the blood clotting protein used to correct their bleeding problems. These illustrate the vital importance of fool-proof screening of blood and blood products. Of course, intravenous drug users are at risk through needle sharing. Other than these means of transmission, no others have been confirmed.

VACCINES AND IMMUNIZATION

The widespread use of immunization with vaccines has been largely responsible for controlling several serious bacterial and viral diseases. However, we must remember that many effective vaccines have not been used widely in developing countries and that moreover, in these areas, diseases caused by various parasites are responsible for causing great misery and many deaths. As you will see later, parasitic infections are very difficult to control by immunization and they present one of the great challenges to immunological science. Before dealing with these, however, we will examine some of the successful bacterial and viral vaccines.

Types of Immunization

Passive Immunization. There are basically two types of immunization, passive and active. Passive immunization involves the transfer to one individual of antibodies formed in another. For example, years ago anti-tetanus serum was made in horses immunized with tetanus toxoid and this was then given to humans to prevent tetanus. Allergic reactions – serum sickness – to the horse protein were often produced which were distressing, and sometimes even fatal, to the patient.

All antibodies used for passive immunization are now of human origin to minimize allergic reactions to them. Passive immunization with antibody gives *immediate* protection, but it does not last very long because antibodies survive in the circulation for only a few weeks and as they break down and are removed, so the protection acquired passively is lost.

Having said this, passive immunization with specific antibodies is used very effectively to protect against tetanus and rabies, and in a similar manner also against the toxins in snake venom. Antibodies against the rhesus blood group antigen are also used in a different way, as we shall see later, to prevent mothers being sensitized immunologically to the rhesus antigens on the red blood cells of their newborn children.

Active Immunization. By this we mean that the individual is intentionally immunized with killed or live microorganisms to induce a state of specific immunity. The protection given by this sort of immunization can, in some cases, be life-long, and even if it is not, it is very easy to boost it by a repeat immunization. You can understand how this works so effectively if you recall the features of a secondary immune response (see Figure 13). Because immunization creates a lot of memory lymphocytes, these can make a very rapid response to infection so that the infection does not cause disease.

The immunity that arises from natural infection is always the best, so vaccines are designed to mimic this as far as possible. However, it is not safe to give live organisms that can themselves cause disease, so they are treated, or attenuated, to make them innocuous but still able to immunize. Unfortunately, killed viruses do not induce very effective immunity when used as vaccines. Although antibodies may be readily induced, effective T cell responses do not occur, largely because proteins from dead viruses do not get presented by MHC class I molecules to activate T-cytotoxic cells. The standard immunization schedule used in the UK is laid out in Table 6.

Immunization schedule		
Vaccine	Timing	To whom given
Mass programmes		
Triple vaccine {Diphtheria, Tetanus, Pertussis} Polio	3 doses at 3 months, 6 weeks later, 6 months later & boosters at school entry and leaving (tetanus and polio only)	Everybody
Measles (& mumps & rubella in some countries)	Second year of life	Everybody
Selective large scale programmes		
BCG	10–14 years of age	Tuberculin-negative individuals
Rubella	10–14 years of age	All girls
Influenza	Annually in the autumn	Elderly, chronically sick
Travellers to developing countries		
Cholera Typhoid Yellow fever	During the month or so prior to travel	
Exposure (occupational or accidental)		
Hepatitis B	Pre-exposure	Health care personnel
	Post-exposure	Neonates of carriers
Rabies	Pre-exposure	Some laboratory and kennel workers
	Post-exposure	Individuals bitten or licked by infected animals

Table 6. Immunization schedule.
Mumps and rubella vaccines are given at the same time as measles vaccine in some countries. In addition to those mentioned here, normal human immunoglobulin and tetanus and polio boosters should be considered for travellers to developing countries.

Efficacy of Vaccines. Smallpox was eradicated by a successful worldwide vaccine programme and poliomyelitis occurs only very rarely (in about two to three per million children immunized where the vaccines are widely used). Rabies virus can now be given safely as a vaccine without the terrible side effects that used to occur when it was grown in rabbits' spinal cord.

Two other examples show the dramatic effect of immunization (Figure 44). Before the Second World War there were up to 75,000 notifications of diphtheria per year in the UK.

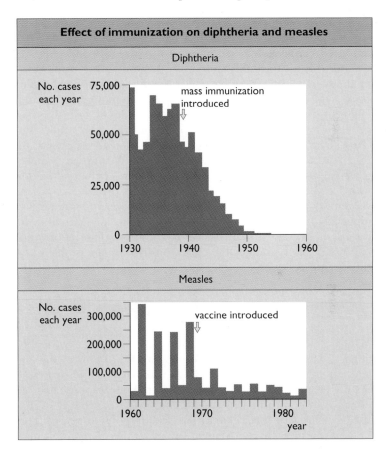

Figure 44. The effects of immunization on diphtheria and measles. As a result of a national immunization campaign started in 1940 in England, diphtheria was effectively eradicated during the next ten years. In England and Wales, a mass vaccination campaign against measles started in 1968 and immediately reduced the number of cases. Unlike diphtheria, however, this vaccination programme has not eliminated measles completely and a small epidemic still appears in a two-yearly cycle.

83

Immunization was introduced in the 1940s and in ten years the disease had been eradicated. The introduction of live attenuated measles vaccine in 1968 also led to a very marked drop in reported cases, although there is still a seasonal pattern evident in Europe. In emergent countries, measles is a major cause of death in children where mass immunization is not available. We should mention that immunization programmes are only effective in controlling disease when almost everyone at risk is immunized. For this reason, immunization should always be carried out, for example with the well-known Triple vaccine, even in areas where the diseases concerned are very rare.

Improved Vaccines. It is very hard to produce safe and effective vaccines for all bacterial and viral infections using traditional methods. However, there have been some very exciting and successful developments through the use of genetic engineering and synthetic protein chemistry. For example, by inserting the genes from dangerous viruses into another relatively innocuous virus, or bacterium, a piggy-back vaccine can be produced. In other cases, recombinant DNA methods have been used to make a vaccine for the hepatitis B virus that is now safely used worldwide, and a similar approach is likely to produce a rabies vaccine. Leprosy and AIDS are two diseases where vaccines are especially needed and, of course, the parasite diseases that we discuss below are a main focus of attention. They, however, because of their complex life cycles, present unique problems to the vaccine designers.

IMMUNITY TO PARASITES

Malaria, other protozoa and various sorts of worms probably affect two billion people worldwide (Figure 45) producing disease and misery on an enormous scale. As with bacteria and viruses, if the organism is in the blood stream, an antibody response may be effective in controlling its spread, and if the parasite is within tissues or growing intracellularly, a T cell response develops. The immunity arising from infection by many of these organisms may not only be effective in clearing the infection but may also provide long-lasting resistance to re-infection. Unfortunately, that is by no means always the case because the host may not become immune after infection for reasons we will explain.

Antibody Response Against Parasites

Individuals with a good IgG response do have protection against blood-borne parasites, such as the trypanosomes which cause Chagas disease. On the other hand, with helminth worms such as trichinella, large amounts of IgE antibodies are produced and a greatly increased number of eosinophils are found in the blood. IgE antibodies can be used to kill parasites with the help of eosinophils, platelets or mast cells through antibody-dependent cell-mediated cytotoxicity (also see type II hypersensitivity).

The major parasites that infect humans		
Parasites responsible	Disease	No. of people affected
Protozoa		
Plasmodium	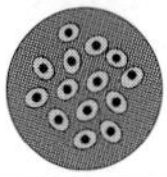 Malaria	350,000,000
Leishmania	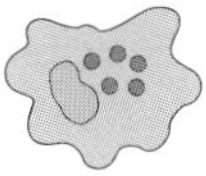 Leishmaniasis	12,000,000
Trypanosoma	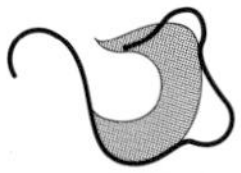 Chagas disease (South America) Sleeping sickness (Africa)	25,000,000
Helminths		
Trematodes (flukes)		
Schistosoma	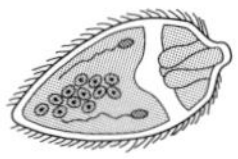 Schistosomiasis	250,000,000
Nematodes (roundworms)		
Ascaris	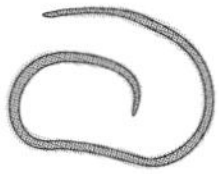 Ascariasis	1,000,000,000
Ancylostoma Necator	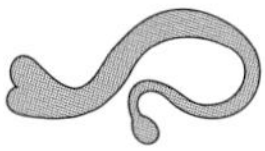 Hookworm	900,000,000
Wuchereria Onchocerca	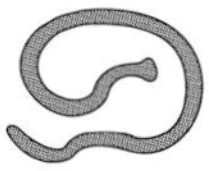 Filariasis (elephantiasis, river blindness)	100,000,000

Figure 45. The major parasites that infect humans.
We cannot know the exact number, but it is estimated that around half the people in the world suffer from some form of parasite infection. All parasites cause some sort of illness or malaise, and many are fatal. The infections they cause represent the major challenge to medical science.

85

The relative functions of antibodies of different types are such that in naturally immune or vaccinated hosts, IgG (and IgA) may provide resistance to infection, whereas IgE antibodies may be necessary for recovery from infection.

T Cell Responses

Although there is little evidence that T-cytotoxic cells are important in resistance to parasites, it is clear that cytokines secreted by T cells *are* very important. They are particularly involved in activating macrophages to kill parasites that are growing intracellularly. It is clear that eliminating worms, for example, needs both antibody and T cell-mediated immune responses to be effective.

Why are Parasitic Infections so Difficult to Deal with Immunologically?

There are many reasons for this and they reflect the fact that these organisms have perfected the art of parasitism and thereby evade the host's immune response. Evasive action takes a number of different forms and those that are best understood are summarized in Table 7. For example, mycobacteria (TB) and histoplasma (a fungus causing lung disease), although not 'typical' parasites, both cause similar lung diseases and both live in macrophages thereby being protected from immune destruction. The African trypanosome (a protozoan) and *Borrelia* (a bacterium) each evade the host's antibody response by changing their surface antigens. In this way they are not susceptible to damage by the antibodies that have been made in response to natural immunization with the parasite. The trypanosome has a remarkable ability when changing its coat antigens to make up to 1,000 different proteins in an ever-changing sequence. You can see how this makes it impossible for the host to make an effective antibody response. As a result, such parasites cause a relapsing or undulant fever. Every successful parasite lives in such a way that it evades those immune mechanisms which are most likely to damage or eliminate it.

All immune reactions depend on the initial recognition of the parasite by the cells of the immune system. The tapeworm echinococcus lives in a hydatid cyst, usually in the liver, quite out of reach of the immune system and thus avoid recognition and attack. Some organisms, as mentioned already, live inside cells and thus escape detection. Others are even more devious and absorb host molecules onto their surface, a good example of this being the schistosome which absorbs red cell lipids, MHC molecules and immunoglobulin fragments, making itself antigenically like the host and therefore invisible to the immune system.

Ways parasites evade attack by immune mechanisms	
Concealment by:	Living inside host cells
	Hiding inside a capsule made by the parasite
	Hiding inside a cyst
	Living in a privileged site from which immune cells are absent
	Mimicry of host antigens
	Acquiring a coat of host antigens
Antigenic variation by:	Mutation of genes coding the antigens
	Programmed expression of only one of many different genes coding the antigens
	Recombination of genes coding the antigens
Immunosuppression by:	Immunologically non-specific means
	Immunologically specific means through compromising actions of macrophages or T cells

Table 7. Ways parasites evade attack by immune mechanisms.

Worms that live only in the lumen of the gut are really outside the body and beyond the reach of attack by lymphocytes and phagocytes. IgA antibodies may be made and secreted into the gut but they do little harm on their own and worms often have a cuticle that prevents antibody binding. Finally, some parasites that do enter the body release large amounts of their own antigens into the circulation which block potentially damaging lymphocytes and antibodies from reacting against the parasites themselves.

Effective Immunity Against Infection
Here you have seen the types of immune response against microorganisms and larger parasites that may prevent or control infection. On the other hand, these infectious agents have a great variety of ways to evade immune destruction. The balance then between host and parasite is dynamic, with both driving the actions of the other.

We must emphasize that all these parasites are very complicated from the immunological point of view: they have many different antigens and it is important to realize that not all immune responses against such complex antigens are effective. This is vitally important in understanding how vaccines work. It is essential that they stimulate a form of specific immunity of exactly the right type directed against the right antigen at the right stage of the infection in order to be effective.

HYPERSENSITIVITY AND ALLERGIC REACTIONS

Hypersensitivity reactions arise from the usual adaptive immune responses and the ways they work depend upon immunological memory for a particular antigen or *allergen*. The intensity of a hypersensitivity reaction often increases with repeated exposure to the stimulating agent. This is very obvious in the case of a drug allergy where it is extremely rare to find an allergic reaction, such as a rash, after only the first course of, for example, the antibiotic responsible for the allergy.

The problem with these reactions is that they are exaggerated or inappropriate forms of adaptive responses, which coincidentally damage one's own tissues in the process of producing the immune reaction which itself is directed to the destruction of the foreign antigen. This damage occurs because the body is either exposed to an excessive amount of antigen or because antibody to it is made in too high a quantity. In special cases, hypersensitivity reactions happen when antibody or T cells are directed against antigens of one's own body, as in the so-called autoimmune diseases. In all these situations the individual is said to be hypersensitive. Hypersensitivity reactions are classified into four types according to their mechanisms (types I, II, III and IV), the first three of which are mediated by antibody, the fourth being antibody-independent and mediated by T cells and macrophages. Antibody mediated reactions occur more quickly after a second challenge with the antigen than those mediated by lymphocytes alone.

ATOPY AND ANAPHYLAXIS (TYPE I)

The clinical conditions embracing asthma, eczema and hay fever are called *atopic* disorders and occur in people who have (usually) a family history of these ailments and who also show very rapid wheal and flare skin reactions when skin tested with the most common inhalent allergens. About 15% of the population in the UK have allergic symptoms, such as hay fever due to grass pollen allergy. The prevalence of allergic disorders, such as asthma and atopic eczema, has increased steadily since the 1960s for reasons that are not clear but which may be associated with environmental pollution. Acute *anaphylaxis* mediated through

IgE-dependent mechanisms is seen with food and drug allergy and also most dramatically in the allergic response to bee and wasp stings.

The first description of the mechanism of the allergic reaction was made by Prausnitz and Kustner in 1921 when it was shown that a serum factor (then called reagin, but later found to be IgE antibody) from an allergic subject could sensitize normal skin. The serum from an individual allergic to fish was injected into the skin of a person who was not allergic and who was then skin tested at that site with an extract of fish – resulting in an immediate wheal and flare response. Interestingly, this only worked with an extract of cooked fish (not raw) which suggests that new antigens are revealed by the cooking. Furthermore, if the second healthy individual ate fish after he had sensitized his skin with an injection of allergic serum, a positive skin reaction was again produced. This shows quite clearly that some food allergens are absorbed undigested into the circulation and can reach the target organ – in this case the skin, and cause a reaction.

Genetics of the IgE Allergic Response in Humans

It has been known for many years that allergic parents have a higher proportion of allergic children than those who are not allergic. A raised concentration of IgE in the blood is also a risk factor. If genetic make-up were the sole factor in predisposition to allergy, one would expect identical twins to suffer similarly. Oddly, the concordance of atopy in identical twins is nearer 50% than 100%, which suggests that environmental factors are also important (Figure 46).

The average person inhales about 1 μg (one millionth of a gramme) of pollen grains each year, which seems an extremely low dose so it is surprising that around 15% of us suffer from hay fever. Studies in mice show clearly that the tendency to produce large amounts of IgE is also under direct genetic control.

Mechanism of Atopy

Immediate hypersensitivity reactions occur following interaction of allergen with specific IgE antibody that has been absorbed onto the surface of mast cells and basophils. This leads quickly to degranulation and the release of pharmacological mediators of inflammation (Figure 47). Because mast cells and basophils are in and underneath the skin and the mucous membranes of the nose, throat, lungs, eye, etc. (Figure 48), these are the places most readily affected by atopic reactions. This first, immediate, phase of the inflammation often leads to cells accumulating nearby as part of the inflammatory response that in turn leads to

89

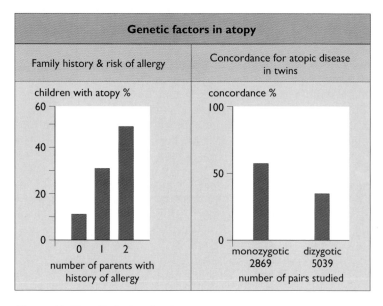

Genetic factors in atopy	
Family history & risk of allergy	Concordance for atopic disease in twins
children with atopy %	concordance %

Left chart:
- y-axis: 60, 40, 20, 0
- x-axis: 0, 1, 2 — number of parents with history of allergy

Right chart:
- y-axis: 100, 50, 0
- x-axis: monozygotic 2869, dizygotic 5039 — number of pairs studied

Figure 46. Genetic factors in atopy.
Left. The incidence of allergy in the population is around 15%. With one allergic parent the percentage of allergic children doubles, and increases further if both parents are allergic. Right. One would expect identical twins to suffer genetically programmed diseases identically. This is not the case and suggests that environmental factors act as important triggering agents.

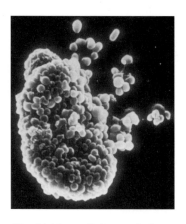
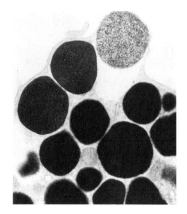

Fig. 47. Mast cell degranulation.
This is the critical event in atopic allergic reactions. These are electron micrographs of a mast cell in the process of releasing its granules as a 'shower' (left). On the right is a section cut through the cell which shows how their structure changes when they have been released: their contents solubilize and cause the inflammatory reactions associated with atopy. Courtesy of Dr TSC Orr.

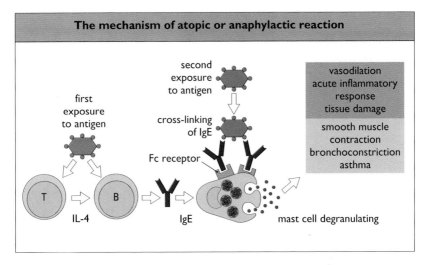

Figure 48. The mechanism of atopic or anaphylactic reaction.
IgE antibodies produced as a result of previous exposure to an antigen (the allergen), such as plant pollen proteins, bind to the Fc receptors on the surface of mast cells, many of which are situated very close to mucosal tissue surfaces. When the allergen is next encountered it binds to the antibodies, cross-links the receptors in the cell membrane and this initiates a series of events that result in the mast cell granules being expelled from the cell and their contents released into the surrounding tissue. Note that basophils also perform in the same way. The mediators of inflammation include histamine and prostaglandins which produce the clinical effects of allergy (also see Figure 39).

further inflammation and other clinical effects some hours later, as in the late phase reaction (LPR) in asthma (Figure 49).

What is interesting here is the effect of drugs. Sodium cromoglycate (Intal®), a drug used for asthma, blocks both the immediate response and also the LPR, which shows that the immediate response is an essential prelude to the LPR. Corticosteroids on the other hand only block the LPR, which in fact is often the most important clinically in chronic asthma. The immediate response is probably caused by *histamine* release, and the LPR probably by *prostaglandins*.

Environmental Factors

Pollutants such as sulphur dioxide, nitrogen oxides, diesel fumes and fly ash may increase mucosal permeability and so enhance the entry of antigen to sensitize by stimulating IgE antibody production. The effect of cigarette smoking seems to vary according to exposure; enhancement of IgE occurs with low level smoking

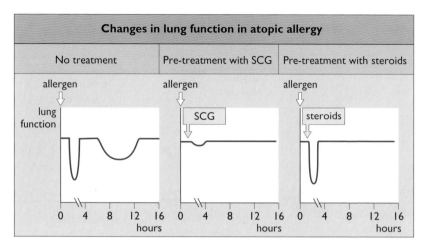

Figure 49. Changes in lung function in atopic allergy.
If an allergic individual inhales the specific allergen then the difficulty in breathing that follows may resolve quite quickly, but it is followed several hours later by another prolonged phase when the lung function is impaired. This is the late phase reaction. Sodium cromoglycate (SCG), a drug taken by many people to control asthma, inhibits both early and late reactions. On the other hand, steroids and drugs that block prostaglandins inhibit only the late phase, not the immediate reaction. This shows that the two phases involve different mechanisms.

and suppression with high levels. Diesel exhaust particulates (DEP) can act as a powerful enhancer of IgE antibody production (Figure 50). They are less than 1μm in diameter and in the air above busy roads can reach levels of 500μg/m^3. The increase in allergic rhinitis (a chronic runny nose) and asthma in the last 30 years parallels an increase in air pollution and diesel exhaust. Thus, environmental pollutants may be contributing to the increase in allergic disease. Remember also that viruses come from our environment, and viral infections of the respiratory tract can also have the same aggravating effects as these other pollutants.

The Beneficial Role of IgE

With all the disadvantages associated with IgE allergic responses, you might ask does IgE actually have a useful function? The answer is that it plays a major role in defence against parasitic worms. If IgA does not effectively prevent entry of the worms or other organisms into the body through the gut, then their contact with IgE-sensitized mast cells will lead to the release of

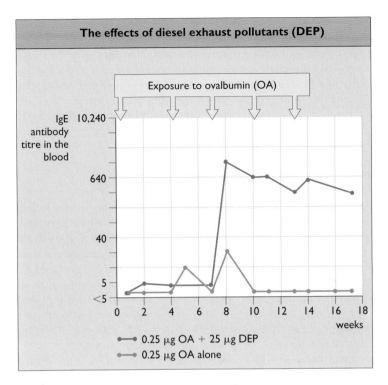

Figure 50. The effects of diesel exhaust pollutants.
Mice who become allergic to ovalbumin (egg white protein) through inhaling it make IgE antibodies just like humans with atopic allergy. The amount (or titre) of antibody they have in their blood is increased if at the time of exposure to ovalbumin they were also exposed to the particles from the exhaust of diesel engines. This suggests why it is that city dwellers (humans) now seem to be more prone to develop atopic allergies. This is just one reason why controlling exhaust emissions is important.

mediators, recruitment of serum factors (IgG and complement) and chemotactic attraction of eosinophils and neutrophils to set up the inflammation as a means of local defence.

When you consider that more than one third of the people in the world have parasitic worm infections, you can understand what a tremendous evolutionary pressure there has been for the development of effective immune mechanisms for dealing with them. IgE and mast cells are the result of that evolutionary pressure, and allergies like those described here are the unavoidable consequence of having this protective immune machinery.

CYTOTOXIC HYPERSENSITIVITY (TYPE II)

There is a large and varied group of diseases and conditions which share the basic common feature of involving IgM or IgG antibodies directed against antigens on the surface of the body's own cells. The effect of these antibodies is to bring about the destruction of the cells in much the same way as foreign bacteria or protozoa are destroyed. Here is another example, as with allergic hypersensitivity, of protective immune mechanisms being involved in damaging anti-self reactions.

Mechanisms of Cytotoxic Hypersensitivity

Once antibody has bound to the surface of a cell there are basically three ways in which the cell can be damaged and killed (Figure 51). The most obvious is that the cell can be phagocytosed because the antibodies bound to its surface engage with Fc receptors on phagocytic cells. This is the process of opsonization described earlier, and in these cases, as with the phagocytosis of bacteria, the activation of the complement system will enhance opsonization and hence phagocytosis. The second way that complement may be involved in cytotoxic hypersensitivity is through initiating direct lysis of the cell coated with antibody. Thirdly, the cells or tissues coated with antibody may be too large to be phagocytosed, in which case the process of extracellular killing (or ADCC) may be initiated. Phagocytes such as neutrophils and macrophages become activated through binding to the antibody-coated target cells and release a combination of lysosomal enzymes, free radicals (reactive oxygen intermediates and, from macrophages only, nitric oxide) and perforins (molecules that make holes in cell membranes) that bring about the lysis and death of the target cell. Note here the similarity with the effect of large granular lymphocytes, or K cells, that also indulge in extracellular killing and are another cell type that may be active in cytotoxic hypersensitivity.

Tissue Susceptibility

One feature of cytotoxic reactions is that different cells are not equally susceptible to the action of the various effector mechanisms. This depends on the amounts of particular antigens expressed on the target cells and to the inherent ability of different targets to sustain damage and repair themselves. In the case of red blood cells, a single hole made by one active complement membrane attack complex is enough to lyse the cell. It requires many more complement complexes to be activated to destroy nucleated cells because of their more active membrane repair mechanisms.

94

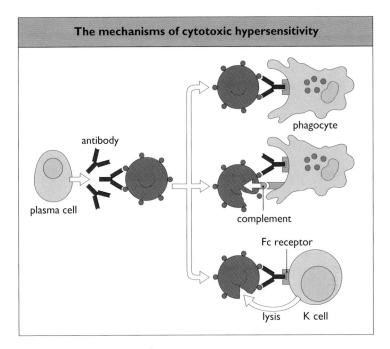

Figure 51. The mechanisms of cytotoxic hypersensitivity.
In this example surface antigens on a red cell stimulate antibody production.
When this binds to the red cells three immune mechanisms may be triggered.
Cells which possess Fc receptors can bind to the red cell via the bound
antibody and lyse it. Such cells are called killer (K) cells. Phagocytes also
possess Fc receptors and engulf the cell. Complement is activated by the
complex of antibody and red cell antigen. Complement lyses the red cell as
described in Figure 36 and opsonizes it for attachment by phagocytes with
complement C3b receptors.

Blood Transfusion

The cells of the blood carry antigens which are the products of
polymorphic genes. This means that some antigens are present
in some individuals and not in others, so a blood transfusion
may actually immunize the recipient against transfusion antigens
that the recipient lacks. This is called *alloimmunization*. It also
occurs naturally by sensitization across the placenta where foetal
red cells can enter the mother's circulation and sensitize her to
antigens [for example, Rhesus (Rh)] that the baby inherited
from the father that the mother herself did not also possess.
Mothers also become sensitized naturally to the HLA molecules
expressed in the foetal leucocytes that enter their circulation
when the placenta breaks down at birth.

95

Blood Group Systems

Red cell antigens are classified into blood group systems, of which the dominant is ABO. Others of importance are the Rhesus, Lewis, Kell and Duffy systems. The importance of a blood group antigen in transfusion depends on the frequency of the corresponding antibody and its ability to lyse red cells *in vivo*. Based on these criteria, the ABO system is pre-eminent.

ABO System. The feature of the ABO system (and all other blood group antigen systems) is that where an individual possesses a particular red cell antigen, the antibody against it is absent. Thus, if a subject is blood group A, he or she will have anti-B antibodies in the circulation, but no anti-A and vice versa. A group O subject will have both anti-A and anti-B antibodies. These so-called naturally occurring antibodies, anti-A and anti-B, only become detectable after the age of 3 months and are probably made in response to A and B antigenic material on bacteria. The A and B antigens are carbohydrates, and as the structure of carbohydrate is much less diverse than those of proteins, you can see that the chances are high of encountering similar antigens on the many bacteria that infect or colonize our body. This is an example of molecular mimicry of antigen where self and bacterial antigens are very similar to each other. This is reflected in animals reared under germ-free conditions where anti-red cell antibodies are much less common than in those reared conventionally.

Rhesus System. Although this is a complex system of several different antigens, it is convenient to classify individuals as either Rh$^+$, 85% of the population or Rh$^-$, 15% of the population, according to the presence or absence of the Rhesus D antigen. It is important to avoid transfusing a Rh$^-$ recipient with cells carrying the D antigen which is the most immunogenic after the A and B antigens of the ABO system. If mismatched red blood cells are transfused these will be coated by antibody, complement will be fixed, leading to red cell lysis causing a severe reaction that can be fatal.

Haemolytic Disease of the Newborn

Sensitization usually occurs at the birth of the first child if the mother is Rh$^-$ and the baby Rh$^+$ because it inherited the Rh antigen from the father. As the placenta breaks down at birth large numbers of Rh$^+$ foetal red cells enter the mother's circulation. If the red cells are not destroyed by antibodies of the ABO system, they remain in the circulation and can induce an anti-Rh IgG antibody response. These antibodies can then cross the placenta during future pregnancies.

The consequences to the foetus of maternal anti-D alloimmunization can vary in severity. Because sensitization of the mother occurs very late in the first pregnancy, her first baby is not at risk. However, subsequent babies are (Figure 52). The foetus may die *in utero* because of severe anaemia due to red cell haemolysis. Some babies can be saved by intra-uterine transfusions, and others can have exchange blood transfusion after birth to minimize further haemolysis and reduce the level of bilirubin (a breakdown product of haemoglobin) which may cause toxic and permanent brain damage (kernicterus).

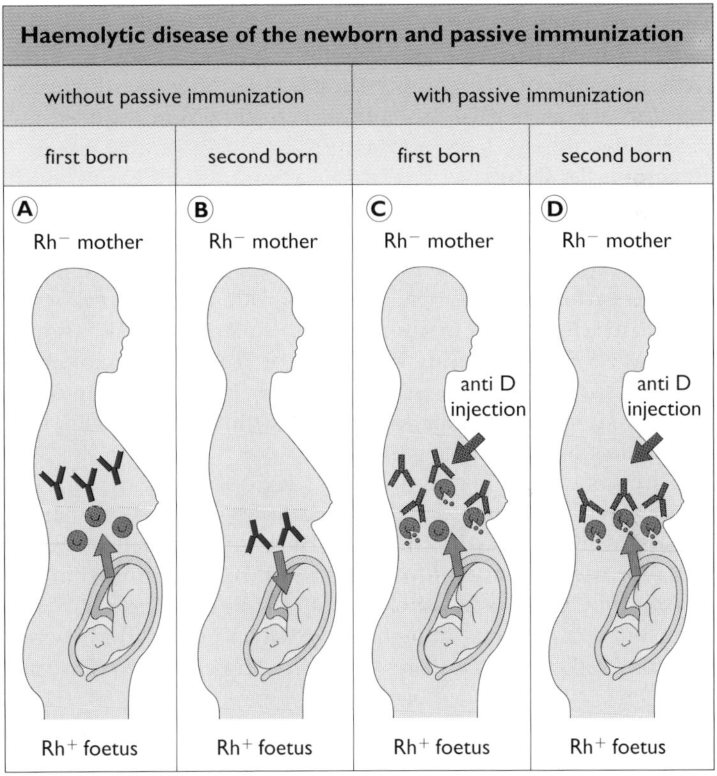

Figure 52. Haemolytic disease of the newborn and passive immunization.
When a Rh⁻ mother is exposed to the red cells of a Rh⁺ baby at birth, she may produce anti-Rh antibodies (A), which will damage a second Rh⁺ baby (B). This can be avoided by injecting anti-Rh antibody at the first birth so that foetal red blood cells are destroyed before they can activate the maternal immune system (C). Thus, the second birth of a Rh⁺ baby will be undamaged (D), although passive immunization of the mother at birth will, of course, be required again in order to protect any subsequent Rh⁺ baby.

Anti-D Prophylaxis. Fortunately, this haemolytic disease of the newborn is now understood, is controllable and can be largely avoided by preventing sensitization of the mother in the first place. This is done by passive immunization (Figure 52). Immediately after the birth of her child, the mother is injected with anti-RhD antibodies. These bind to any foetal erythrocytes that have entered her blood stream and bring about their destruction, thereby preventing them sensitizing her immunologically. The next baby to be conceived develops in an environment free of these damaging antibodies. This treatment is one of the triumphs of obstetrics and immunology and can potentially eliminate anti-D haemolytic disease of the newborn. It is now standard treatment for all mothers at risk. The incidence of new cases of maternal Rh sensitization has fallen dramatically in the UK since the early 1970s when this treatment was introduced.

Reactions To Drugs

If a drug binds to the surface of blood cells it can provoke an antibody response against the drug itself and also the cell membranes onto which it is bound. Examples of this are found in the destruction of red cells, causing haemolytic anaemia, following administration of penicillin or sulphonamides. We should emphasize that reactions like this are relatively uncommon amongst the many people who need to use these drugs. In those who do suffer such a hypersensitivity reaction, the problem subsides after they cease taking the drug.

Thrombocytopenic purpura (involving destruction of platelets by antibodies) was seen in the past with the sedative drug, Sedormid, which was withdrawn because of these adverse reactions. In the case of Sedormid purpura, fresh serum from the patient will lyse normal platelets, but only in the presence of the drug and complement, thus showing that an interaction between the drug and platelets is necessary, as is complement, to cause the lysis.

Reactions to Tissue Antigens

There are many diseases where an individual who was otherwise healthy begins to make antibodies that damage a particular tissue or cell type. These are the so-called autoantibodies and the diseases are known as autoimmune diseases. Autoantibodies alone are not responsible for the pathology of all autoimmune diseases, for in many cases we know that T cells are also involved. However, there is good evidence that autoantibodies are very important in the progression of some autoimmune diseases, and we will describe some of these in this section.

We should remind you in passing that autoantibodies are made as natural components of the immune system, and it is only in particular diseases that they cause pathology. It is clear that the damaging autoantibodies have a relatively high affinity for their target antigen, they are made in sustained large amounts and are often of the IgG class. Natural autoantibodies on the other hand are IgM antibodies, usually of low affinity, and present in small amounts. We are largely ignorant of the stimuli that give rise to the immune activation leading to autoimmune diseases but we are beginning to understand that apparently unrelated infections may be very important in some cases. Because we do not understand the origin of autoimmune diseases, we refer to them as being idiopathic. Clearly, there are genetic risk factors, the most notable being MHC class II genes for many diseases but, again, it is not certain how these operate. The next decade will undoubtedly reveal to us how many of these diseases originate.

Thyroid and Endocrine Tissues. The thyroid is one of the tissues most often affected by autoantibodies which are directed against cells and molecules on and in the gland itself. This can lead to damage or destruction and as a result cause diseases such as Hashimoto's thyroiditis (Figure 53). The concept of organ-specific autoimmunity was introduced more than 30 years ago by Ivan Roitt and Deborah Doniach who demonstrated the existence of anti-thyroglobulin antibodies using a simple agar precipitation test.

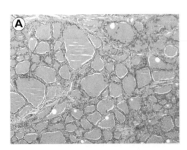

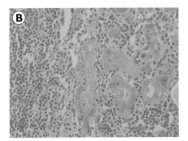

Figure 53. The thyroid gland in Hashimoto's thyroiditis.
The large follicles are a conspicuous feature of the healthy thyroid gland – they contain the colloid material essential to the normal functioning of the thyroid (A). In inflammatory diseases of the thyroid, blood mononuclear cells infiltrate the gland and destroy its structure. In advanced cases, little of the normal structure survives, the thyroid being almost entirely replaced by inflammatory cells which may become organized into lymphoid follicles (B). Compare this with the structure of an activated lymph node (Figure 16). These follicles are a marker of sustained local immune activation. Courtesy of Professor Neville Woolf.

Other endocrine tissues can also be the targets for autoimmune attack by antibodies and the range of effects (Table 8) include diseases of the stomach and adrenal glands that involve antibodies to gastric parietal cells and adrenal cortex, respectively. More recently, autoantibodies to the insulin-producing islet cells in the pancreas have been detected in the serum of patients suffering from insulin-dependent diabetes mellitus (IDDM). In all these diseases, the immune damage to the endocrine tissue upsets the hormonal balance of the body. Drugs and replacement hormones such as insulin are required to control the metabolic imbalance that follows. There is considerable interest in the possibility of transplanting the appropriate cells to replace those damaged in the disease; currently there is great effort being made to transplant pancreatic cells in diabetics.

Autoimmune endocrinopathies	
Thyroid disorders	Hashimoto's thyroiditis
	Primary myxoedema
	Grave's disease (thyrotoxicosis)
Gastric disorders	Gastritis with/without pernicious anaemia
	Autoimmune antritis
Other disorders	Insulin-dependent diabetes mellitus
	Addison's disease (autoimmune adrenalitis)
	Autoimmune hypogonadism and adrenalitis
	Autoimmune hypophysitis
	Autoimmune hypoparathyroidism
	Vitiligo

Table 8. Autoimmune endocrinopathies.
These autoimmune diseases affect primarily one organ or tissue and are characterized by the presence of T cell and B cell (autoantibody) reactivity against antigens restricted to that tissue alone. Some of these diseases may occur together in families or individuals.

Basement Membranes and Goodpasture's Syndrome. A number of patients with nephritis (inflammation of the kidneys) are found to have antibodies directed against the kidney glomerular basement membrane (Figure 54). These are IgG antibodies and can generally fix complement. The resulting inflammation (nephritis)

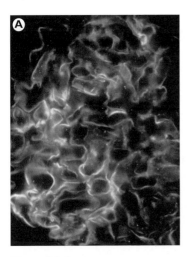
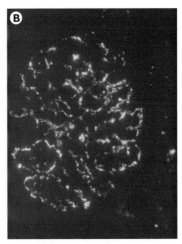

Figure 54. Immune complexes in the kidney.

Immune deposits of antibody, or antibodies and antigen, can form or be deposited in the kidney in several different ways. They are most easily detected, as here, by using anti-immunoglobulin antibodies labelled with a fluorochrome that is visualized under a fluorescent microscope. (A) In Goodpasture's syndrome, antibodies against an antigen that is part of the basement membrane bind all along the convoluted shape of the membrane. (B) On the other hand, complexes of DNA and anti-DNA antibodies deposit in isolated spots on the membrane or in association with the cells of the kidney mesangium in systemic lupus erythematosus

causes necrosis (death) of the glomerulus which becomes clogged with fibrin, badly damaging the filtration capacity of the kidney. It was noticed by Goodpasture (hence the syndrome named after him) that some patients with nephritis also had lung haemorrhage. This is due to the antigenic similarity of the basement membranes of the glomerulus and the lung, so that antibodies directed to the one will bind to the other and also cause damage.

Some years ago Goodpasture's syndrome was fatal; more than 90% of patients dying because of kidney or lung damage. When it was shown that autoantibodies were responsible for the tissue damage, attempts were made to suppress antibody production with drugs such as corticosteroids and immunosuppressive agents. The results were not impressive. However, the management of this disease was transformed by plasmapheresis or 'laundering' of the blood. It was argued that if the antibody was actually removed, the patient would improve – as indeed they do. Blood is removed from the patient, the cells separated and washed, the plasma discarded, and the cells put back into the patient with fresh plasma.

Plasmapheresis is now used in of other diseases where circulating autoantibodies or toxins are the main cause of the tissue damage. The results are very encouraging in the treatment of some cases of myasthenia gravis, rhesus haemolytic disease and cryoglobulinaemia, but not as successful as in Goodpasture's syndrome.

Myasthenia Gravis. In stimulating muscle contraction the normal nerve impulse involves the release of acetylcholine (ACh) from the nerve ending which diffuses across the neuromuscular junction to bind to ACh receptors on the muscle endplate. In myasthenia gravis there is extreme muscle weakness as a result of antibodies binding specifically to the ACh receptor on the surface of the muscle endplate. This makes the impulse less effective in triggering the muscle (Figure 55). This is due to two reasons. First, the antibody binds to the ACh receptor and blocks the action of ACh itself and second, the bound antibody fixes complement which actually destroys the receptor sites. People with myasthenia gravis, not surprisingly, have weak muscles that tire easily and can eventually become paralysed.

Drug treatment is aimed at blocking acetylcholinesterase, the enzyme that breaks down ACh, so that there is more available to trigger the muscle. There are also a number of immunological treatments such as immunosuppression, thymectomy and plasmapheresis that can be helpful. It is probable the T cells also contribute to the pathology, but in ways not yet understood.

Blood Cells

We have already described the special haemolytic anaemias that occur when drugs become attached to the surface of red cells. However, there are also several diseases where autoantibodies are formed against the antigens that normally exist on red cells, platelets and leucocytes. For example, antibodies against antigens on red cells cause the complement-dependent destruction of red cells and hence a clinical anaemia. In some cases these are obviously formed as a consequence of infection, a good example being streptococcal infections that, in a few unlucky people, may cause not only an anaemia of this sort but also kidney disease and rheumatic heart disease. Each depends upon cross-reactive antibodies whose production was first stimulated by the bacteria.

The destruction of blood platelets leading to thrombocytopenia has been mentioned, again in the context of drug reaction, but in many cases anti-platelet antibodies appear for no obvious reason. There are also several diseases in which autoantibodies against lymphocytes are produced, although we do not know with assurance the extent to which they contribute to direct pathological effects.

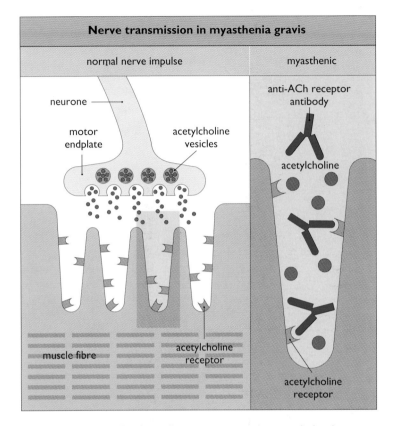

Figure 55. The mechanisms that prevent nerve transmission in myasthenia gravis.
Normally, a nerve impulse passing down a neurone which arrives at a motor endplate causes acetylcholine-containing vesicles to fuse with the cell membrane and release their acetylcholine (ACh). This diffuses across the neuromuscular junction and combines with ACh receptors on the muscle causing the ion channels in the muscle membrane to open and the muscle to contract as a result. In myasthenia gravis, antibodies are made against the receptor which impair its ability to bind ACh, leading to poor muscle function and sometimes paralysis.

IMMUNE COMPLEX HYPERSENSITIVITY (TYPE III)

When antigen combines with antibody in the body, immune complexes are formed which initiate a series of events which normally culminate in the elimination of the antigen through phagocytosis by cells of the monocyte-macrophage system. In some cases, however, the reaction is exaggerated and leads to a tissue-damaging inflammatory response. When localized in a

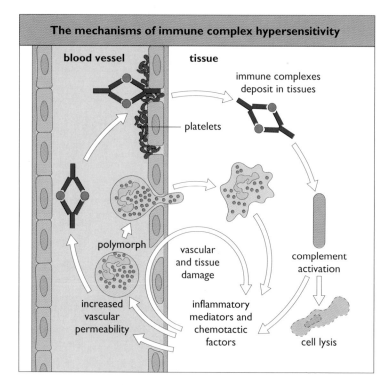

Figure 56. The mechanism of immune complex hypersensitivity.
When antigen and antibody are deposited in tissue together as an immune complex, complement may be activated. The inflammatory mediators which are produced increase vascular permeability, thus further increasing deposition and attracting polymorphs by chemotactic factors. These cells cause vascular and tissue damage which cause more mediators to be produced. Complement can also cause direct tissue damage by lysing cells to which antibody or complexes are attached. (More details of the processes of cell migration are in Figure 5.)

particular tissue this response is called an Arthus reaction. When spread through the body it is called serum sickness (Figure 56). However, it is important to remember that the formation of immune complexes is basically a natural and protective process. For example, after any meal the level of immune complexes in the blood is high and this represents a normal physiological response. It is only when the body is exposed to an excess of an antigen over a long period of time, such as with a microbial organism or other foreign antigen, or in autoimmunity to the body's own tissues, that the immune complexes cause damaging inflammation (Table 9).

Varieties of disease caused by immune complexes		
Origin	Antigen	Sites of complex deposition
Persistent infection	Microbial antigen	Infected organs, kidney
Autoimmunity	Intrinsic self-antigen	Kidney, joint, skin, arteries
Inhaled material	Extrinsic environmental antigen	Lung

Table 9. Varieties of disease caused by immune complexes.
This is a simplification of very complicated disease processes to indicate the major organs affected in different types of immune complex diseases.

General Mechanisms of Immune Complex Hypersensitivity

When large amounts of complexes are formed the phagocytes may become overloaded. This causes the prolonged circulation of the complexes and they deposit in vulnerable sites such as the glomerulus of the kidney. Red blood cells play a part in the removal of complexes through their complement receptors (CR1) which bind immune complexes and transport them to the liver and spleen where complexes and receptors are removed by the resident phagocytes. Each red cell has about 700 of these receptors, and in immune complex disease the number of receptors per cell falls steadily, further impairing the efficiency of the immune complex removal machinery.

The key is to appreciate that although immune complexes may persist in the circulation for a long time, simple persistence is not usually harmful in itself. Problems only start to occur when they deposit in tissues.

Immune complexes trigger a variety of inflammatory processes. First, their interaction with complement leads to the production of the anaphylatoxins C3a and C5a, which in turn trigger basophils and mast cells to release histamine and other inflammatory substances. Second, chemotactic agents are produced for neutrophils and monocytes. Third, compounds that activate lymphocytes and other phagocytic cells are also generated. The mixture of inflammatory events caused by these agents leads to increased vascular permeability, which in turn causes the accumulation of cells and fluid in the tissues. Immune complexes can also interact with platelets through their Fc receptors causing them to aggregate and form a clot or thrombus; this further increases vascular permeability through the release of vasoactive amines. These various mechanisms are summarized in Figure 56, which emphasizes that in all these reactions blood vessel walls are an important site of complex deposition.

Arthus Reaction

If soluble antigen is injected into the skin of humans or animals who have high levels of specific antibodies in their blood, an oedematous red swelling appears after 4–10 hours which usually disappears by the next day. Microscopically, numerous polymorphonuclear leucocytes can be seen where the injection was given. The antigen, in combination with antibody, deposits in the walls of local blood vessels, binds complement and causes the cascade of inflammation mentioned above. The Arthus reaction can be blocked by depleting the body of neutrophils or complement, which demonstrates their importance in the process.

Hypersensitivity Lung Diseases

The Arthus reaction itself is a rather artificial procedure but it demonstrates the mechanism of damage in, for example, respiratory (lung) diseases. When antigen is inhaled by a patient who has high levels of circulating IgG antibody, immune complexes form on the mucosal surface (air side) of the lung where they cause tissue damage (Figure 57). Breathing difficulties occur over a similar time course to the Arthus reaction in the skin; symptoms start 4–10 hours after exposure and gradually resolve over the next 24 hours. The lung is immunologically different from the skin in that, as a result of the mucosal inflammation, the lung becomes 'over-sensitive' for many days.

Farmer's lung is due 'to antibodies produced in response to the inhalation of spores from mouldy hay and extracts of these microorganisms give a positive Arthus skin test when injected into the skin of affected individuals. A similar lung problem occurs in Pigeon Fancier's disease, and in a variety of occupational lung diseases such as Cheese Washer's disease, Furrier's lung and Maple Bark Stripper's lung, in each of which antigen is directly inhaled. The antigens are different but the mechanisms are the same.

In allergic bronchopulmonary aspergillosis a mixture of hypersensitivity and allergic reactions are seen; patients have an IgE-dependent allergic (type I) reaction to *Aspergillus fumigatus* and asthma, as well as an immune complex (type III) hypersensitivity that together cause lung damage. In addition, the organism remains in the lung to provide a chronic antigenic stimulus.

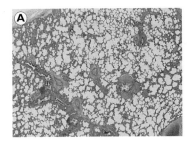

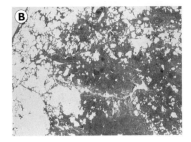

Figure 57. Farmer's lung disease. Damage caused by immune complexes.
When a farmer inhales the spores of the mould *Micropolyspora faeni*, IgG antibodies are produced which can be detected in the blood. On further exposure, the mould antigen and antibody form immune complexes in the lung which fix complement and activate an inflammatory cascade leading to an influx of cells. This in turn leads to considerable destruction of the air spaces, alveoli, with inflammation and fibrosis. Above is shown a section of normal lung with intact air spaces. In Farmer's lung, below, one can see considerable cell infiltration and destruction of the alveoli.

Serum Sickness

It was once commonplace to use horse antibodies against the tetanus organism to protect people who were at risk from tetanus, having cut themselves in, for example, the garden or sports field. A similar use of serum was also taken to protect against diphtheria. In both cases, the antibodies were given as passive immunization, and in conjunction with antibiotics were reasonably protective. However, the recipient would almost always make large amounts of antibody against the foreign horse serum proteins so that if the therapy was ever repeated enormous amounts of immune complexes were formed. The results were sometimes catastrophic. This is the phenomenon of serum sickness and the events that follow the first exposure to the foreign serum proteins are illustrated in Figure 58.

Reactions very like serum sickness can also occur as a result of allergic reactions to antibiotics. In these conditions the immune complexes deposit in a whole range of tissues in the body causing a generalized severe systemic illness. To cause inflammation, the complexes have to be the right size. If they are too large they are removed immediately by macrophages; if too small they continue to circulate, are only slowly removed and do not cause inflammation. The right-sized complexes localize through a change in vascular permeability, probably following from platelet aggregation and the release of 5-hydroxytryptamine or through complement-mediated degranulation of mast cells and

107

basophils releasing histamine, leukotrienes and platelet activating factor. These mediators enable the complexes to sieve through the endothelial cell layer and deposit in the basement membrane of the skin, joints, kidneys and heart. If there has been only a single injection of antigen, once antibody synthesis has reached an adequate level, antigen is cleared from the circulation and the patient usually recovers. It is repeated exposure to the antigen that causes the greatest problems.

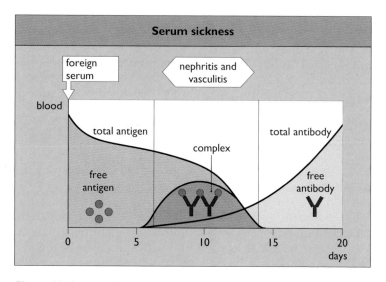

Figure 58. Serum sickness.
In humans or animals, after foreign serum has been injected, antibodies are made against the proteins of the injected serum and can be found in the blood after about five days. These antibodies bind to the foreign serum proteins to make immune complexes, and it is then that the symptoms of serum sickness appear. They are caused by the complexes becoming trapped in the blood vessels and the kidneys where they cause vasculitis and nephritis, respectively. Later, the amounts of antibody increase and the amount of antigen decreases; then symptoms subside. This shows you that the ratio of the concentration of antibody to the concentration of antigen determines the biological effects – pathology in this case – of the immune complexes.

Immune Complex Kidney Disease

Many cases of glomerulonephritis are associated with the presence of immune complexes in the glomerulus, as illustrated in Figure 54.

Immune complex deposits can be seen in some cases following infection with certain strains of streptococci and also in some types of malaria. They are found, especially in the kidney, in some people after therapy with a whole range of different drugs. Bone marrow transplant patients who suffer graft-versus-host disease also have complexes in their kidneys. Complexes can also be detected in the renal arteries of patients who have chronic hepatitis B infections and also in those infected with other viruses such as lymphocytic choriomeningitis virus which can cause a true immune complex glomerulonephritis. In many diseases, the complexes in the kidney do not seem to cause any significant damage and we can view their presence there as part of the physiological processes that remove immune complexes from the circulation.

Systemic Lupus Erythematosus. Immune complex nephritis is common in patients with systemic lupus erythematosus (SLE) (Figure 54B). Immune deposits of DNA and anti-DNA antibodies can be detected in the glomerulus, but it is difficult to find complexes in the plasma. The likely explanation is that DNA binds non-specifically to the glomerular basement membrane first and this then captures circulating antibody to form the complex *in situ*. This actual sequence can be seen in mice injected with bacterial endotoxin. This causes the widespread release of DNA which then binds to the collagen in the basement membrane of the glomerulus. If anti-DNA antibody is now given, it will bind to the DNA to form complexes in the kidney. Thus, we know of two ways at least by which complexes lodge in tissues: either they are pre-formed in the circulation or they build up sequentially in the place where they cause the damage.

In SLE, immune complexes can also deposit in the skin and the blood–brain barrier where they respectively initiate inflammation that causes the characteristic lupus skin rash and neurological complications. We do not know why such large amounts of anti-DNA antibodies are made in SLE, but it may well be that this autoimmune disease is initiated by an infection of some sort.

DELAYED-TYPE HYPERSENSITIVITY (TYPE IV)

All the forms of hypersensitivity discussed so far depend upon antibodies for their damaging mechanisms. Although T cells are involved in many cases in helping antibody production they do not participate in the disease-damage associated with the first three types of hypersensitivity. However, delayed-type hypersensitivity is mediated by T cells alone and it is they that initiate tissue damage. It is called delayed because the reactions are slow to express themselves after antigen challenge. It is obviously associated with T cell protective immunity but does not always coincide with it. The T cells necessary for producing the delayed **109** response are cells which have become specifically sensitized to the particular antigen by previous encounter, and they act by recruiting other cell types to the site of the reaction. Mostly it appears to be $CD4^+$ Tdth cells (also known as TH1 cells) that secrete selective cytokines such as IL-2 and IFN-γ that cause the typical lesions of delayed hypersensitivity. The action of these cells is probably controlled by other $CD4^+$ T cells (known as TH2 cells) that secrete IL-4 and IL-10, so you can imagine that the balance between protective and damaging immunity partly reflects the way in which different lymphocyte populations interact with each other.

There are three forms of delayed hypersensitivity: contact hypersensitivity and tuberculin reactions (the first two) occur within 72 hours of applying or injecting the antigen whereas granulomatous reactions (the third) develop over weeks. The granulomas are formed by aggregation and proliferation of macrophages and may then persist for weeks or months. As with the antibody-dependent types of hypersensitivity which can overlap, the situation is similar with delayed-type hypersensitivity. The different types of reaction may overlap or even occur sequentially following a single antigen challenge.

Allergic Contact Dermatitis and Eczema

Contact hypersensitivity is primarily an epidermal phenomenon in distinction to tuberculin reactions which take place in the dermis, but its basic mechanism typifies delayed-type hypersensitivity. (Figure 59). The *Langerhans cell* is the principal APC in contact hypersensitivity and is also very important in another skin disease – atopic eczema. The reaction is characterized by redness of the area and small blisters which develop at the site of contact. In Europe the most common agents are small molecules (haptens) such as nickel, chromate, and certain hair dyes, and in the USA poison ivy and poison oak are also very important.

Only a very small proportion of people exposed occupationally to a sensitizing antigen will develop sensitivity and the time taken for it to develop varies with the antigen. Bricklayers exposed to chromate in cement may take 10 years or more to become sensitized, whereas hairdressers who develop sensitivity to *p*-phenylene diamine in hair dyes may do so after only a few months of exposure. Some haptens such as dinitrochlorobenzene (DNCB) will sensitize almost all individuals.

Some sufferers with skin eczema find that sunbathing may improve this condition. This is almost certainly because the ultraviolet (UV) in sunlight either destroys or prevents the Langerhans cells in the skin from presenting antigens.

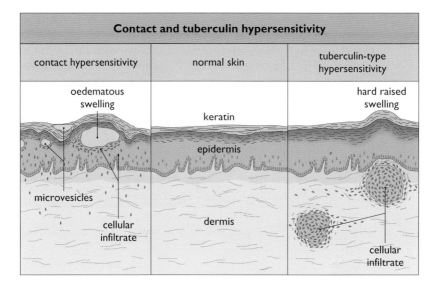

Figure 59. Contact and tuberculin hypersensitivity.
The responses in contact hypersensitivity and tuberculin reactions are both mediated by cells. However, the site of inflammation is different in that cells infiltrate the epidermis in contact hypersensitivity, causing the epidermis to be pushed outwards. A characteristic feature of skin contact allergy is the formation of microvesicles and oedema within the epidermis with redness and small blisters seen on the skin. In tuberculin-type hypersensitivity the cells mainly infiltrate the dermis. This results in a hard raised swelling (induration) on the surface of the skin and redness over the site of the tuberculin skin test.

Unfortunately, others who have eczema may have an opposite reaction to sunlight – they develop an itchy rash, and indeed, people who are not atopic can also become sensitive to UV light.

Tuberculin-type Hypersensitivity

Patients who have recovered from tuberculosis or who have been immunized with BCG have T cells that recognize tuberculin. If tuberculin (a purified extract of the tuberculosis organism) is injected into the skin, T cells migrate from the capillaries and the cellular infiltrate extends outwards reaching its greatest extent 48 hours later. The induration (hard, raised swelling) around the site of the injection is quite different to the oedema (weal) and flare seen in atopic skin reactions (Figure 59).

Macrophages are probably the main APC in tuberculin-type hypersensitivity reactions and they start to accumulate around small blood vessels in the dermis at 12 hours, increasing up to 72 hours (Figure 60). As the tuberculin lesion develops it may

111

become granulomatous because the antigen persists in the tissues. We must emphasize that this type of reaction, although clinically associated with sensitivity in tuberculosis, can occur to a great variety of microbial, and non-microbial antigens. Its basic value in protective immunity is that it represents a local reaction that is designed to contain and, if possible, destroy the infectious agent. The fact that it does not always achieve this is a tribute to the devious life-style of the organism that initiated the reaction.

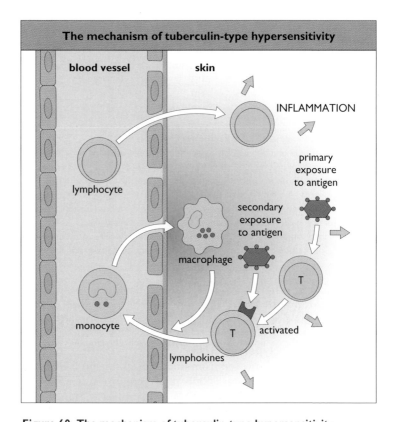

Figure 60. The mechanism of tuberculin-type hypersensitivity.
When tuberculin is injected into the skin of someone already immune to it, there is considerable cell migration. Lymphocytes migrate from the blood vessels and accumulate in the skin and at the same time macrophages and Langerhans cells migrate from the epidermis. By 48 hours there is a cellular infiltrate present in all areas, especially the dermis. Cells in the overlying epidermis express MHC class II molecules and ulceration can occur. Classically, the skin surface shows a nodular erythematous area – the hallmark of the tuberculin skin test.

Granulomatous Hypersensitivity in Tuberculosis and Leprosy

This is clinically the most important form of delayed hypersensitivity causing much of the tissue damage in diseases which involve T cell immunity. Examples of this are the cavitation, caseation and general toxaemia seen in human tuberculosis and in the granulomatous skin lesions of leprosy.

The microscopic appearance of a granuloma is quite different from that of the tuberculin-type reaction where the response is self-limiting (because the soluble antigen becomes degraded) rather than being due to persistence of a living, multiplying antigen. The characteristic cells in granulomatous hypersensitivity are the epithelioid cell, a large flattened cell with increased endoplasmic reticulum and sometimes called *Langhans giant cells* (not to be confused with the Langerhans cells discussed earlier). Giant cells have several nuclei ranged around the periphery of the cell.

An immunological granuloma has a core of epithelioid cells and macrophages, sometimes with giant cells. In TB, for example, the central area may be necrotic with complete destruction of all cellular structure (Figure 61). The macrophage/epithelioid core is surrounded by a cuff of lymphocytes and there may also be fibrosis which is a physiological response to wall off the site of persistent infection. Granulomas in tuberculosis can occur throughout the body wherever

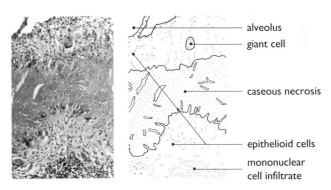

alveolus
giant cell

caseous necrosis

epithelioid cells
mononuclear
cell infiltrate

Figure 61. Tuberculous lung.
In tuberculosis there is granuloma formation in the lung, skin and other affected organs. The reaction is frequently accompanied by external fibrosis. The histological appearance is typical of a granulomatous reaction, with a central caseous (cheesy) necrosis. This is surrounded by an area of epithelioid cells containing multinucleated giant cells, and the whole area is one of increased cellular activity.

mycobacteria exist, and not just in the lung with which the disease is most often clinically associated.

Granulomas of another type can also be produced by non-antigenic particles such as inorganic talc which macrophages find totally indigestible, but these granulomas do not have the cuff of lymphocytes surrounding the core.

In leprosy, protective immunity depends solely on T cells and macrophages with antibodies playing no part. The spectrum of responses in leprosy varies between those people who respond well to the leprosy mycobacterium ('tuberculoid leprosy') and those with no response ('lepromatous leprosy'). In between these two extremes lies borderline leprosy. We mentioned before the role of T cells making different cytokines in delayed-type hypersensitivity. Here it seems that if T cells making IL-2 and IFN-γ are dominant, the tuberculoid response occurs whereas if T cells making IL-4 and IL-10 predominate a lepromatous response happens. In leprosy we now know that not only CD4$^+$ T cells are important, but also CD8$^+$ T cells can contribute to its pathology and to the natural regulation of disease.

Borderline reactions occur either naturally as a sign of the disease or following drug treatment of pre-existing leprosy where areas of the skin become swollen and inflamed because of sensitivity to the antigens of *M. leprae*. This process of inflammation and cell infiltration also occurs in the peripheral nerves and is a most important cause of nerve destruction in this disease. The lesion in borderline leprosy is typical of granulomatous hypersensitivity.

Autoimmune Diseases and Delayed-type Hypersensitivity

There are many diseases in man and animals which show delayed hypersensitivity and most are due to infections. The pathogens present a persistent chronic antigenic stimulus, stimulating a continual release of cytokines from sensitized T cells with the resulting accumulation of large numbers of macrophages. However, there are many autoimmune diseases in which infectious microorganisms have not been identified as the cause but which, nonetheless, show exactly the same type of responses dependent upon T cells and macrophages that damage tissues. In fact, the great majority of autoimmune diseases involve demonstrable T cell reactivity to autoantigens. We have already mentioned many human autoimmune diseases, so you will be familiar with this fact already. It is clear that humans and animals have the same sorts of autoimmune diseases. Here we will describe some animal experiments that have been very important in enabling us to interpret disease mechanisms in humans.

Experimental Autoimmunity. It is a general finding that an animal immunized in an appropriate way with cells or extracts of a particular tissue will develop an autoimmune lesion in that same tissue. The importance of T cells can be demonstrated in several different ways: (i) by their reactions to tissue-specific antigens *in vitro*; (ii) by their involvement in skin test sites where microscopically the response looks just like a tuberculin reaction; and (iii) by the ability of purified T cells to adoptively transfer disease to an otherwise healthy animal. We should stress that the last of these three, cell transfer, exemplifies an experimental approach that has been absolutely crucial in unravelling the workings of the immune system. By comparing the effects of transferring different types of cells, and antibodies too, from immune to normal (unimmunized) animals, many basic mechanisms have been explained. These range from the demonstration that lymphocytes are the agents of immunity, through T cell–B cell cooperation, to the effects of different profiles of cytokine release in different tissues. Such experiments are, of course, impossible and unethical in humans.

Experiments of this sort have highlighted some exciting possibilities for the therapy of autoimmune diseases. At this point we will just say that T cells are clearly important in the development of multiple sclerosis, thyroiditis, some forms of arthritis and diabetes, amongst many other diseases. In general, CD4$^+$ Tdth (TH1) cells making IL-2 and IFN-γ seem to promote pathology and others (making IL-4 and IL-10) (TH2) seem to regulate it. A role for transforming growth factor-β (TGF-β) is now recognized in regulating T cell activity in autoimmunity. It is generally believed that the inappropriate activation of T cells is central to the initiation of at least *some* autoimmune diseases. You will recall that not all self-reactive lymphocytes are destroyed during the development of the immune repertoire and it is the cells that escape elimination that later do the damage. Obviously there are very special circumstances surrounding their activation and although the picture is not yet complete it is clear that genetic factors (especially the MHC type) are important and that environmental factors (most often ill-defined infection) contribute as well to inducing autoimmune disease.

TRANSPLANTATION

With increasing understanding of the MHC, sophisticated immunosuppression regimes and skillful surgery, more and more different organs and tissues can be transplanted. These include kidney, heart, liver, lungs, bone marrow, skin and, of course, cornea and heart valves. Transplantation biology has grown into an enormous subject, particularly because of its successful clinical applications and great potential for further success.

The immune basis of the rejection of tissues transplanted between genetically unrelated individuals has been recognized for many years. Despite this, immune reaction is the major cause of graft loss in man. The immune mechanisms underlying rejection are not fully understood, but it is clear that the situation is complex, often involving antibodies, $CD4^+$ and $CD8^+$ T cells working in concert. Graft rejection has all the characteristics of an immune response. An individual will reject transplants from all genetically non-identical donors. If a graft, for example skin as shown in Figure 62, is taken from one inbred mouse and transplanted to one of a different strain, it is rejected. A second transplant of another graft from the same sort of donor is rejected more quickly, whereas one from a second type of donor behaves like the first graft transplanted. So, graft rejection displays specificity, diversity and memory, and the most important antigens determining rejection are MHC molecules (HLA in man and H-2 in the mouse).

Immune Responses to Transplants
Cell transfer experiments have shown us in an unequivocal way that T cells are essential for graft rejection and this is reflected in the fact that humans and animals who are born without a thymus, and hence have no T cells, or who are immunosuppressed, do not reject transplants. If you recall our discussion of the MHC, you will remember it is a highly polymorphic system. Indeed, it has to be like this to fulfill its natural function of antigen presentation, but it is this very polymorphism and the fact that T cells are designed to react to MHC molecules that makes it so important in transplantation. This is where the MHC got its name: small differences in the structure of MHC molecules between individuals are avidly recognized by T cells in the graft recipient and reacted against. So you can see that rejection of foreign tissues is biologically unavoidable and, furthermore, that the cells that provide protective immunity to infectious microorganisms are the same cells that destroy transplants. It is for this reason that the MHC products that exist on all cell membranes are often referred to as 'transplantation antigens'.

As well as T cell-mediated reactions, both animals and humans make an antibody response accompanying graft rejection. If a further similar graft is given, hyperacute (very rapid) graft rejection may occur because of antibody-mediated reactions against the grafted tissue. This is a problem that makes the selection of second grafts for patients who have rejected their first grafts all the more difficult. Further, the usually benign process of blood transfusion may induce antibodies that would subsequently

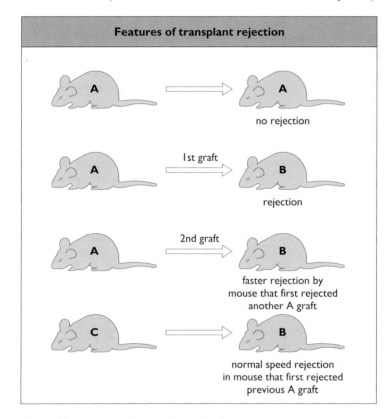

Features of transplant rejection

A → A
no rejection

A → 1st graft → B
rejection

A → 2nd graft → B
faster rejection by mouse that first rejected another A graft

C → B
normal speed rejection in mouse that first rejected previous A graft

Figure 62. Features of transplant rejection.
This is illustrated by what happens to skin grafts transplanted between mice of different inbred strains. Each strain is genetically different from the others, but all the animals in one particular strain are identical to each other. When skin is transplanted between mice of the same strain (A), there is no rejection, but grafts exchanged between mice of any two different strains (A and B) are rejected. When a second graft is transplanted onto a mouse that has already rejected a first graft, it is rejected much more quickly provided it comes from the same donor as the first; if from a different donor (C) it is rejected in the normal time for a first graft. This shows you that graft rejection is under genetic control and that autoimmune rejection of grafts does not occur. Importantly they show you that graft rejection has all the features of an adaptive immune response: rejection reactions are diverse (all foreign grafts are rejected) and specific and display memory.

damage grafted tissue. For tissues that do not become vascularized, rejection of any sort is rarely a problem. A good example of this is in corneal grafting where most grafts are accepted even though there may be an HLA mismatch between the donor and the recipient. Cartilage is similarly accepted in the face of HLA incompatibility. With bone and artery, MHC mismatching is not so important as the tissues are largely free of cells and just provide a scaffold for the cells of the host to colonize.

Survival of Grafts

The ideal foreign graft would come from someone with an *identical* HLA make-up to the recipient, so that there will be no rejection. The best candidate here would be an identical twin but, of course, one is only rarely available. It is normal therefore to transplant immune tissues from relatives or unrelated donors. Often, considerable effort is made to find donors who are very similar to the recipient with regard to their HLA 'antigens' (remember the enormous polymorphism of the system) to minimize the incompatibility and hence limit the strength of the rejection reaction. The probability of finding an HLA completely identical, but unrelated, donor is negligible, but fortunately matching for the class II genes (effectively the DR genes) may be greatly beneficial (Figure 63A). Class I matching is also important, so in practical terms the best matched graft available is usually used. Tissue typing is the name given to the procedures used to identify HLA genes and their class I and class II products.

The HLA system, however, is not the only gene system to code for transplantation antigens. In fact there are many donor antigen systems that are only really important in the transplantation of free cells rather than tissues, bone marrow and pancreas islet cells being examples. Although it is rare for these to be matched for other tissues, it is the case that the ABO blood group system is vitally important for survival of all transplants with a connected blood supply. Thus, kidney donors and recipients are always matched for compatibility for this system. You would be right to assume that ABO antigens are expressed on many cell types apart from red blood cells. Note, however, that because red blood cells do not express HLA, tissue typing is not required for blood transfusions!

Immunosuppression

In practical terms, wherever tissues (apart from blood) are transplanted from one person to another it is essential to suppress the immune response of the recipient, no matter how perfect the HLA matching has been. Many different ways have been tried for this but all those in widespread use have the disadvantage that they are immunologically non-specific. The consequence is that there is sometimes a difficult balance between immunosuppressing enough to prevent rejection while still leaving the immune system functioning adequately to deal with infection. The goal, not yet achieved, is to find a way of generating donor-specific immunosuppression that leaves the immune machinery otherwise completely intact. The major approaches to immunosuppression are described below.

Purine Analogues. 6-Mercaptopurine (6-MP) is an example of a drug that acts as a cell poison by inhibiting nucleic acid synthesis. This is a very toxic compound and in an effort to make it less so, azathioprine was developed which when metabolized by the liver is converted to 6-MP. The targets for such compounds are the lymphocytes but as they also block all actively dividing cells their use can reduce all the white cells of the blood, cause hair loss and damage the liver and lining of the gut.

Corticosteroids. Corticosteroids are made naturally by the cortex of the adrenal glands and are natural regulators of immune cell function in healthy people. This is one example of the relationship between the endocrine and the immune system. Corticosteroids can also be synthesized chemically and used as drugs with a multiplicity of different biological functions in the body, and although very effective at this, their exact mode of action in suppressing graft rejection is still not fully understood. As well as their anti-inflammatory and immunosuppressive properties, these compounds stabilize cell membranes, alter the way cells travel around the body (cell traffic), and can slow down cell division. It is not known which function is particularly beneficial in preventing graft rejection. In atopic allergy, we should mention that corticosteroids, especially those not absorbed across mucosal surfaces, can be very beneficial.

Cyclosporin. This is a very impressive compound that was isolated as a peptide from a fungus – *Tolypocladium inflatum*. What is so valuable is that cyclosporin preferentially affects dividing, but not resting T cells, and also inhibits cytokine production. Resting T cells which carry memory for immunity to infections are not affected. Cyclosporin is thus a very powerful immunosuppressive compound, but it has the disadvantage of also being toxic to the kidney. This makes it somewhat difficult to use in renal transplantation, where it is important to make the diagnosis between graft rejection and nephrotoxicity due to the drug. **119**

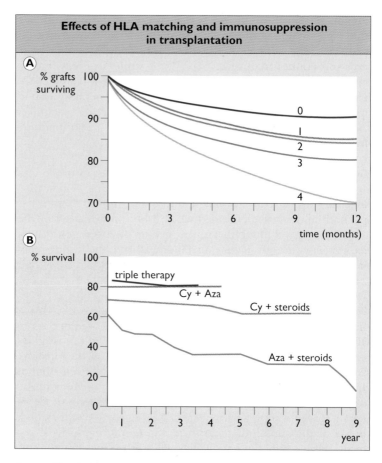

Figure 63. Effects of HLA matching and immunosuppression in transplantation.
A. The effect of matching for HLA-B and DR in cadaver kidney transplant patients treated with cyclosporin. The curves show survival rates of grafts incompatible for 0 to 4 HLA-B plus DR antigens (adapted from Opelz, 1987). B. This shows the survival of heart transplant patients treated with different immunosuppressive regimes involving azathioprine (Aza), cyclosporin (Cy) and steroids in various combinations. Courtesy of Mr T English.

The usual way to avoid this is to use it in combination with other drugs – so called combination therapy – allowing each to be used in smaller doses than would be necessary when used alone (Figure 63B).

This drug revolutionized transplantation in the 1980s through its greatly superior efficacy as an immunosuppressant compared with cytotoxic drugs and steroids. As you can imagine, there is great competition to isolate other natural peptides, or make synthetic peptides, that would be even more effective. A newer compound called FK506 is another example of the family of cyclosporin-like drugs. Because of its effects on activated T cells, cyclosporin is also sometimes used to control autoimmune diseases, one other set of situations aside from transplantation where immunosuppression may be needed clinically.

Irradiation. Not widely used, but selective irradiation of major lymph nodes can be very effective in controlling transplant rejection.

Immunosuppressive Antibodies. There are numerous examples of particular antibodies being immunosuppressive (Table 10). Although some that show great promise are still very much in the experimental stage, others such as anti-lymphocyte serum (ALS) have been widely used in combination with drugs to good effect.

Donor Antigen. You would expect that a previous exposure to an HLA antigen that is the same as one expressed on a graft would make the recipient more likely to reject it. While this is true generally, there are situations where it enhances graft survival. Although the general experience may vary from country to country and from hospital to hospital, recipients who have had many blood transfusions seem to derive a benefit from this, although they cannot be given a graft if they have antibodies against its HLA class I antigens. It is thought that some HLA class II antigens, expressed on the white cells in the transfused blood, induce a form of protective immunity. This encourages scientists to look for selective ways of 'specifically immunizing' graft recipients to make them better able to prevent rejection by natural immunological means.

Types of Transplant

The kidney was one of the first organs to be transplanted and many thousands of successful operations have now been done throughout the world. The success rate is now in the region of 85–90% functioning grafts at one year. Recipients who reject a kidney can be maintained on a dialysis machine and successfully re-transplanted later.

Heart and heart–lung transplantation is now almost equally successful in centres with experience, with graft survival of approximately 80% at one year (Figure 63B). This is a very impressive figure because there is no possible artificial support system (as with the kidney) to maintain the circulation beyond the first few hours if rejection does occur. 121

Immunosuppressive antibodies and transplantation		
Antibody	Target	Effects
Anti-lymphocyte serum/globulin (ALS)	T cells	General immunosuppression
Campath-1	T cells	Lytic destruction of cells (with complement)
Anti-CD3, CD4 or CD8	T cells	Stops activation of T cells
Anti-IL-2R	Activated T cells	Selective suppression of activated cells after their encounter with antigen
Anti-LFA-1	Lymphocytes	Prevents effective immune cell co-operation, and leucocyte interaction with vascular endothelial cells
Anti-MHC class II	Activated lymphocytes	Prevents lymphocyte activation
Enhancing antibodies	MHC antigens on the graft	Limits sensitization of the host

Table 10. Immunosuppressive antibodies and transplantation.
These are largely experimental antibodies, except that ALS has been widely used in humans and campath-1 is an example of an antibody first discovered through animal experiments that, through genetic engineering, is now available in a potent form suitable for use in humans. The actions of most antibodies are not completely worked out, but they might also be valuable in other situations where T cell activity needs to be controlled, such as autoimmune diseases.

The liver is less immunogenic than other organs and it less readily induces rejection. This is illustrated in animals where some grafts survive without any immunosuppression, and in humans where HLA matching is not needed, although immuno-suppression is essential.

The cornea is a natural *privileged site* and not connected to the immune system. What is unusual about the healthy cornea is that it has no arteries, capillaries or veins or lymph vessels, and is not rejected because lymphocytes do not reach it. Only when the cornea is vascularized, which can happen when it is inflamed, is rejection likely. In this situation, immunosuppression becomes crucial.

PREGNANCY

It is strange to consider the foetus as a 'graft' but it does contain paternal antigens that are foreign to the mother. In the human placenta, lymphocytes of the maternal blood circulate in intimate contact with the placenta, which is a foetal tissue, yet the foetus is not rejected like a transplant by the mother. Probably an important factor is the absence of both conventional class I and class II MHC molecules on the placental tissue which make it less susceptible to immunological attack.

Maternal factors are also important. You can imagine that it would be immunologically convenient if the mother was specifically tolerant to the paternal antigens in the foetus but there is little evidence for this. There *is* evidence for a generalized immunosuppression of immunity during pregnancy as shown by reduced delayed hypersensitivity skin tests to tuberculin, reduced antigen-induced lymphocyte stimulation, and reduced lymphocyte reactivity between mother and foetus or between parents. However, these responses are not absent, merely reduced. Hormones secreted by the placenta and changes in corticosteroid levels probably contribute to the immunosuppression. Basically we are largely ignorant of why the mother does not reject her foetus and whether immune mechanisms have any role in the natural processes of birth.

CANCER

If tumours really expressed antigens that were quite different from those of the surrounding normal tissues, it would be expected that immune reactions would be able to destroy them. This idea has a long and illustrious history and it led Burnet, and others, to develop the idea that immune surveillance by lymphocytes was responsible for recognizing and reacting effectively against the foreignness of tumour antigens. Without doubt this is an elegant hypothesis, although it has been difficult to examine experimentally. In some animal systems these mechanisms may operate, but support for effective surveillance from human tumour biology is hard to find.

What makes most tumours different antigenically is a quantitative rather than a real qualitative change in the expression of some particular molecules which are, in some cases, otherwise found only during foetal, but not adult life (so-called oncofoetal antigens). Immune responses may be made against these, in the same way that they are made against virally-coded antigens on **123** tumours induced by viruses. It is estimated that 75% of all human tumours are induced by chemical (environmental) carcinogens and 20% of tumours in women and 10% in men are linked to virus infections. Quite how these different tumour-inducing agents work is not known in detail, but in many cases so-called *oncogenes* are activated which in turn activate other genes that lead to the unrestrained division of the cells.

IMMUNOSUPPRESSION AND TUMOURS

Patients who have been transplanted, and who by necessity are immunosuppressed with drugs, have an increased incidence of tumours, especially in the lymphoid system (lymphomas). They also more frequently have tumours of the skin and vaginal cervix that are probably related to virus infections. AIDS patients, who are naturally immunosuppressed, have an increased incidence of non-Hodgkin's lymphoma and Kaposi's sarcoma.

This pattern of tumour incidence in immunosuppressed patients is different from that in the rest of the population. One explanation may be that the drugs reduce the effectiveness of T cell-mediated activity against cells that are made malignant by persistent infection with viruses such as cytomegalovirus (CMV) or the Epstein-Barr virus (EBV) that causes glandular fever. This may also be the case in AIDS, where T cells are reduced in number by the disease, and infection by microorganisms and parasites increases.

Malaria and Burkitt's Lymphoma

Malaria produces an immunosuppression which reduces immune responses against B cells that have been infected by EBV. In normal people without malaria, such B cells transformed by EBV are killed by T-cytotoxic cells, although latent virus infection will persist subsequently throughout life. In adolescents, however, the mild immunosuppression caused by malaria may allow a single clone of B cells to escape destruction and develop into a lymphoma. This is a clinical example of how one infection (malaria) may affect the way another (EBV) progresses: the epidemiological association of malaria and lymphoma was recognized long before EBV itself was discovered.

Immune Responses Against Established Tumours

When a tumour grows in an immunocompetent host it is assumed that is has evaded recognition and elimination by the immune system. However, such tumours are often infiltrated by lymphocytes that are themselves activated. Thus, it seems that tumours evoke an immune response that may not to be sufficient to prevent tumour growth. This may be explained by induced immunosuppression and the sheer magnitude of the antigenic load. Suppression is probably caused, in part, by tumours inducing the production of cytokines that are immunosuppressive. We also refer to the phenomenon of metastatic insufficiency, by which it is meant that the number of tumour cells shed from a primary tumour into the blood stream is far in excess of the number of cells that finally grow into metastases or secondary tumours. This tells us that the host *is* able to deal successfully with some but not all tumour cells. That the human immune system is capable of limiting tumour growth to some extent is shown by concomitant immunity, where small tumours become infiltrated by lymphocytes and disappear while large tumours are unaffected, and the latency of secondary tumours that only grow after the removal of their primary tumour. There is also the observation that chemotherapy is more effective *in vivo* than *in vitro* suggesting that there is also a useful endogenous anti-tumour response that can be stimulated under the correct conditions.

Immunotherapy with LAK Cells
Because the immune system cannot destroy large tumour masses, it is important to reduce the tumour load by surgery or radiotherapy before attempting immunotherapy. Expanding the lymphocytes which can infiltrate a tumour by treatment *in vitro* with IL-2 and then re-injecting them into the host does seem to be partly successful in some patients with malignant melanoma. Such lymphokine-activated killer (LAK) cells have also been given to other cancer patients with some promising but varied results (Figure 64).

Hybridoma Antibodies as Magic Bullets
The successful clinical application of novel or conventional therapeutic products in cancer is crucially dependent upon their selective delivery to the right place in the body. Exciting developments in monoclonal antibody technology may now make this possible. If it is possible to identify a specific tumour antigen then a 'magic bullet' of specific antibody coupled to a toxin such as ricin might be an effective therapy (see Figure 35). This has been achieved experimentally and may yet be possible in the future in humans.

Bispecific monoclonal antibodies have been made which recognize two different antigens. One Fab arm recognizes the tumour and the other recognizes molecules such as drugs or toxins, thus specifically focussing them onto the tumour cells **125**

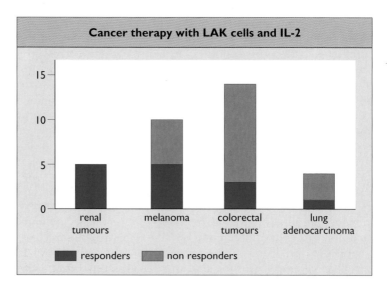

Figure 64. Cancer therapy with LAK cells and IL-2.
LAK cells are produced by incubating a patient's lymphocytes with IL-2 *in vitro*. This activates and transforms the cells and makes them more effective at killing tumour cells *in vitro*. When these cells are returned to the patient they came from, they appear to aid in the destruction of the tumour. In this illustration, the numbers of patients responding to therapy with LAK cells plus IL-2 are shown. Note that this therapy apparently is not equally effective against all types of cancers.

and killing them. The use of bispecific antibodies to carry effector cells to tumours also offers other treatment possibilities. Such molecules may activate lymphocytes localized in the tumour to release therapeutically important cytokines. In concept this is much the same as using gene transplantation to make tumour cells express cytokines like IL-2 that will activate lymphocytes.

In an attempt to improve the activation of targetted effector cells, antibodies capable of reacting with three distinct antigens (trispecific antibodies) have been made by linking different Fab fragments together. For example, one may be directed against a tumour antigen while the others respectively combine with molecules like CD3 and CD28 that are molecules on effector T cells. These antibodies are intended to bring immune cells and their targets together more effectively than happens naturally.

Other Treatment Possibilities
Other novel molecules with clinical potential have been made by joining non-antibody molecules to fragments of antibodies either by biochemical means or by linking their genes by genetic

engineering. Either way, the chimaeric or hybrid molecules usually consist of antibody-binding domains of tumour reactive antibodies linked to toxins or cytokines (such as TNF-α) which are either directly toxic to the tumour, or can activate lymphocytes at the site of the tumour. So-called *superantigens* of bacterial origin have been linked to anti-tumour antibody fragments in the belief that such constructs both concentrate lymphocytes in the tumour and enhance their killing activity.

The antibodies for tumour therapy of this sort are directed against tumour molecules, such as tumour-specific antigens, oncofoetal antigens (e.g. carcinoembryonic antigen) and receptors for epidermal growth factor or transferrin.

Antibody Fragments as Imaging Agents
Some of the value in the clinical use of antibody fragments comes from their small size that makes them particularly effective at penetrating tissues. This gives them advantages over whole antibody molecules in both therapy and and also in imaging. Imaging is used to locate tumours and other lesions, and it usually involves injecting radio-isotopically labelled antibody fragments directed against an antigen which is unique to the target or present in it in relatively high amounts. Binding of the antibody to the target is imaged using specific photographic techniques to detect the emitted radiation.

THERAPEUTIC CYTOKINES TO STIMULATE OR SUPPRESS IMMUNITY
Our ability to clone lymphocytes and to isolate and clone their genes has enabled us to produce large amounts of pure cytokines. There has been an explosion of information on the diversity of cytokines, their structure, genes and receptors. Our appreciation of some of their physiological roles has increased greatly and hence their relevance to disease processes and their likely therapeutic value have become apparent.

New cytokines are discovered with great regularity. Much effort is invested in answering such basic questions as, what stimuli influence the induction and expression of cytokine genes, what cells do cytokines interact with, how do they interact, what are their effects on the cell and what soluble factors in the body modify their activity? On the clinical side, interest continues in the roles all these play in the pathogenesis of all classes of immunological diseases. We have mentioned the importance of cytokines in many places already. Here, we collect together a few observations and potential uses of cytokine interventions to stimulate or suppress immunity.

In infectious diseases and malignancy, strategies for enhancing the activity of specific cytokines could be very useful. These could involve the development of new ways to induce the expression of cytokines within particular tissues or to target cytokines to specific sites in the body. In the second context it is interesting to note that genetically engineered antibody–cytokine fusion molecules have already been developed with the aim of targeting TNF-α and IL-2 to tumours.

In contrast, in other situations such as autoimmune disease or inflammatory disorders, the inhibition of certain cytokines might be desirable. Recent developments have suggested that one approach to this would be to use particular cytokines themselves. For example, IL-10 exhibits an impressive ability to inhibit the production by CD4 T cells and macrophages of both inflammatory cytokines (IL-1, IL-8 and TNF-α) and those inducing cell mediated cytotoxicity (IL-2, IFN-γ).

There are several other ways that inhibition of cytokines might be achieved (Figure 65). These include inhibiting the synthesis of cytokines or cytokine receptors by drugs, the blocking of cytokine receptors with specific antagonists or cytokine receptor

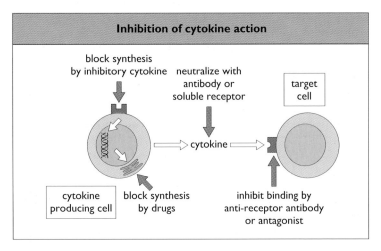

Figure 65. Inhibition of cytokine action.
Although our knowledge of the role of cytokines in health and disease has greatly increased, our attempts to clinically exploit this information is limited largely to the administration of recombinant cytokines. It would obviously be an advantage if we could selectively influence the production, distribution and interaction *in vivo* of individual cytokines with their cellular receptors or with target organs. In this figure we portray various procedures which might be of value in inflammatory disorders. These approaches have been shown to work in experimental systems, but are not yet widely used clinically.

antibody fragments, or the neutralization of cytokines by specific monoclonal antibodies or soluble receptor molecules. It is exciting that the therapeutic value of anti-cytokine antibodies and soluble cytokine receptors in the management of autoimmune diseases and transplant rejection is currently receiving active attention. Clinical experiments show that anti-TNF antibodies may be very effective in patients with septic shock due to infection with Gram-negative bacteria and in controlling some symptoms of arthritis.

Finally, we should mention that some treatment schedules may combine several of the therapeutic approaches we have referred to. For example, TNF-α is being used to enhance the expression of the CEA antigen on colon tumours, thus improving the targetting to this tumour of anti-CEA monoclonal antibodies.

NUTRITION AND IMMUNITY

As we have mentioned, immunodeficiency can be caused by inherited defects, drugs and irradiation, or can be acquired secondarily to a variety of other diseases. Worldwide, nutritional disorders are the most common cause of immunodeficiency: they have been calculated to affect more than 400 million people.

Nutritional Status
It is not only the quantity of food that is important for good nutrition; quality is crucial. Food crops grown in poor soil may be deficient in minerals and trace elements. If the crop is sprayed by pesticides or other chemicals, these can enter the food chain and have further damaging effects on metabolic and immunological processes. The quantity of food is, of course, important too – but we are all aware that undernutrition is rare in the West. Malnutrition can occur also because of poor digestive processes due to gut parasites, enzyme deficiencies, malabsorption, and lack of stomach acid which impair the proper functioning of the gut. There is in fact a multiplicity of other interacting factors that lead to malnutrition and subsequent infection. These include poverty, poor sanitation, lack of health education, sociocultural deprivation, all adding to the difficulties of obtaining adequate nutrition.

In addition to carbohydrate, fat and protein which are building blocks for the body, many other constituents are needed for normal biochemical processes. Mineral trace elements are very important in this respect. There are several hundred metalloenzymes that need trace elements such as zinc, iron, selenium, chromium and copper in order to function properly. In addition, minerals are needed for the anti-oxidant activity of a number of other enzymes such as glutathione peroxidase or superoxide dismutase. The importance of minerals is far outweighed by their apparently normal low level in blood. We can see that many metabolic functions can be significantly changed by subtle changes in nutrition.

Mineral deficiency must be contrasted with the gross changes in protein energy malnutrition (PEM) (Figure 66). Immunodeficiency occurs in PEM and if nutritional deficiency is present during foetal life, the effects on immunity can be severe, long-lasting, and life shortening.

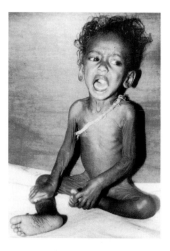

Figure 66. Protein energy malnutrition.
This 13-month-old child shows the gross wasting and wrinkled skin which is characteristic of protein energy malnutrition.

Immune Function and Malnutrition

Many aspects of immune function can be affected by malnutrition (or, indeed, overnutrition in some cases). To give one example that you have seen already, phagocytic cells like neutrophils recognize foreign microorganisms and kill them through activation of complement, release of chemotactic factors, attachment, phagocytosis and an increase in metabolic activity. Several steps in this pathway are affected in PEM, with phagocytosis and intracellular killing of bacteria being notably reduced. Another example in Figure 67 illustrates how the amounts of protective antibody induced by immunization with measles vaccine are reduced in malnourished children.

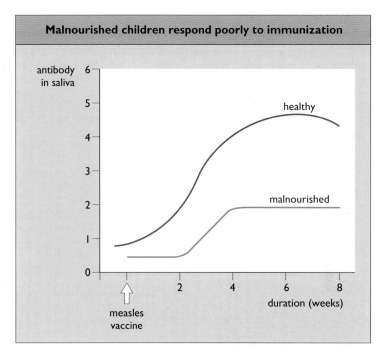

Figure 67. **Malnourished children respond poorly to immunization.**
Here, the effectiveness of measles vaccine is measured by its ability to induce
anti-measles virus antibody which, in this case, is measured in saliva.
Malnourished children make less antibody than healthy children – they also
make antibody more slowly.

Human Importance

The alteration of immune function in nutritional disorders is
important to everyone, but especially to the elderly and to
patients in hospital. Although immune dysfunction occurs early
in malnutrition, it can be corrected and immunological tests
carried out both *in vitro* and *in vivo* can be used as sensitive
assays to detect changes in the nutritional state. One important
clinical strategy depends upon the fact that the response to
immunization can be improved even by short-term nutritional
supplementation given before and after vaccination.

Future Prospects

As the end to our account of the immune system, this is an
example that shows you how the immune system depends upon
and interacts with the other physiological systems of the body.
We hope we have persuaded you that this system is not only vital
to your well-being but also a worthy subject for study. To

complete our story we have gazed into the crystal ball and have put together some predictions in Table 11 of new understanding, achievements and therapies that we anticipate in the last decade of the twentieth century.

Hot tips for the millennium	
Fundamental advances	
Antigen processing	Mechanisms
Antibodies, TCR, MHC	Complete genetic description
Inflammation	Biology of cell interactions, functions of adhesion molecules
Clinical and therapeutic advances	
Autoimmunity	Anti-TNF antibodies suppress inflammatory autoimmunity
	Cytokines and their receptor antagonists suppress disease
	Anti-lymphocyte antibodies (e.g. Campath-1) suppress lymphocytes
	Tolerance from autoantigens swallowed or inhaled
	Vaccines based on TCR molecules to induce suppression
Tumours	Vaccines for viral-induced tumours (e.g. papilloma virus)
	Effective targetting of drugs to tumours using antibodies
Infectious diseases	Development of new vaccines for malaria and other parasite diseases
	Improved adjuvants exploiting knowledge of antigen processing mechanisms
Transplantation	Humanized animal organs and tissues for xenotransplantation
	Donor-specific immunosuppression by graft antigens
	Transplantation of haemopoietic stem cells
Immunodeficiency	Growth factors to rescue deficient marrow

Table 11. Hot tips for the millennium.

GLOSSARY

Acquired immunity: an immune reaction involving lymphocytes that display the features of specificity, diversity, memory, and self/non-self recognition.

Acute phase proteins: liver-derived serum proteins that are produced during the early stages of an inflammatory response.

Adhesion molecules: cell surface molecules involved in the direct binding of one cell to another, or to the substrate, e.g. ICAM.

Affinity: a measure of the binding strength between two molecules, e.g. an antigenic determinant (epitope) and an antibody-combining site (paratope).

Allele: one of several alternate forms of a gene at a single locus that controls a particular characteristic.

Allergen: an antigen that induces an allergic type I (IgE-mediated) hypersensitivity reaction.

Alloimmunization: the process by which one individual becomes immunized against the transplantation antigens of another individual, as may occur through organ transplantation.

Anaphylaxis: an immediate type I hypersensitivity reaction, triggered by IgE-mediated mast cell degranulation causing vasodilation and smooth muscle contraction. The reaction leads to shock and may be fatal.

Antibody: a molecule produced and secreted by lymphocytes in response to antigen, which has the particular property of combining specifically with the antigen which induced its formation.

Antigen presenting cell (APC): a cell (e.g. a macrophage, dendritic cell or B cell) that processes and presents antigen fragments on MHC class II molecules to CD4$^+$ T cells. (This is the classical definition of an APC, but the term is sometimes used for any cell that similarly presents antigen on MHC class I molecules to CD8$^+$ T cells.)

Antigenic determinant (epitope): the part of an antigen with which an antibody or a T-cell receptor molecule interacts.

Antigen: a molecule that binds specifically to antibody or T-cell receptors.

Apoptosis (programmed cell death): a mode of cell death which occurs under physiological conditions and is controlled by the dying cell itself.

Atopy: clinical manifestation of type I hypersensitivity (IgE-mediated allergy) including allergic rhinitis (hay fever), eczema, asthma and various food allergies.

Autoimmune disease: a disease in which specific reactions of the immune system against self tissues or antigens causes or contributes to the initiation or progression of the disease.

B cell: a lymphocyte that has matured in the secondary lymphoid tissues and which has immunoglobulin on its surface as a receptor for antigen.

Basophil: a polymorphonuclear leucocyte that has receptors for IgE antibodies and which may contribute to allergic (type I hypersensitivity) reactions.

Chemokines: a family of diverse molecules that are chemoattractants and activators of inflammatory cells.

Chemotaxis: increased directional movement of cells in response to a concentration gradient of chemotactic factor(s).

Chimaeric antibody: an antibody that has been engineered (at the level of the gene or the protein) in some way so that it is composed of parts originating from different species.

Class switch(ing): the process by which a B cell undergoes V-C gene rearrangement to express a new heavy chain isotype without altering the specificity of the antibody produced.

Clone: a family of cells or organisms having a genetically identical constitution (hence cloning: making a clone).

Complement: a group of serum proteins involved in the control of inflammation, the activation of phagocytes and the lytic attack on cell membranes.

Complementarity determining regions (CDRs): the sections of an antibody or T-cell receptor V region responsible for antigen or antigen–MHC binding.

Cytokines: general term for soluble intercellular signalling molecules, including the interleukins, interferons, colony stimulating factors and tumour necrosis factors.

Cytotoxicity: the processes whereby a cell is killed either by another cell or by chemical means.

Delayed-type hypersensitivity (dth): immune reaction important in dealing with chronic infection which has a characteristically slow appearance when the specific antigen (e.g. tuberculin as a test for tuberculosis) is injected into the skin. Classically associated with the reactions of CD4+ T cells.

Dendritic cells: antigen-presenting cells present in lymph nodes, spleen and at low levels in blood, which are particularly active in stimulating T cells.

Eosinophil: a granulocyte present at less than 5% of peripheral leucocytes, containing granules of cationic proteins which can modulate an inflammatory reaction. Important in atopic allergic reactions and control of parasitic infections.

Epitope: an antigenic determinant q.v.

Gene recombination: the process by which separate pieces of different genes or gene segments are brought together to make a new gene.

Gene segment: a discrete piece of germ-line DNA that contributes to the structure of a functional gene.

Germ-line DNA: the DNA inherited through the gametes from each parent.

Germinal centre: structure within lymph nodes or spleen populated mostly by proliferating and memory B cells.

Haplotype: a set of alleles (genes) present on one parental chromosome.

Hay fever: an allergic (type I hypersensitivity) reaction to environmental antigens (e.g. pollens, house dust) that causes inflammation to the mucous membranes of the eyes, throat and lungs causing irritation, sneezing and breathing problems.

Histamine: a major vasoactive amine released from mast cell and basophil granules.

HLA: the human major histocompatibility complex.

Hybridoma: cell line created by fusing two different cell types, usually lymphocytes, of which one is a tumour cell.

Idiotope: a single antigenic determinant on an antibody or T-cell receptor V region; collectively, several idiotopes are an idiotype. (Anti-idiotype: an antibody against an idiotype.)

Imaging: a process where an antibody labelled with a radioactive isotope is injected and its location in the body revealed with a so-called gamma camera from the outside; used to localize tumours with the aid of an anti-tumour antibody.

Immune complex: the product of an antigen–antibody reaction which may also contain complement components.

Immune surveillance: a process that is thought to involve circulating lymphocytes constantly surveying and reacting against small changes in self body cells arising from mutation or damage and which might be the signs of malignancy.

Immunoassay: a specific laboratory procedure to quantify a substance by use of a specific antibody against it.

Immunocompetence: the ability of the immune system or its individual lymphocytes to react in an immunologically specific way.

Immunoglobulins: alternative name for the family of proteins that are antibodies.

Inflammation: a tissue response to injury or other trauma characterized by pain, heat, redness and swelling. The response consists of altered patterns of blood flow, an influx of phagocytic and other immune cells, removal of the foreign antigen, and healing of the damaged tissue.

Innate immunity: natural, non-specific host defences.

Interferons (IFNs): a group of mediators which increase the resistance of cells to viral infection, and act as cytokines. IFN is also an important immunological mediator.

Interleukins: molecules made by leucocytes involved in signalling between cells of the immune system.

Internal image: a site on some anti-idiotypic antibodies (Ab2) that binds to the antigen-binding site of the antibody (Ab1) and mimics the structure of the original antigen.

Killer (K) cells: a group of lymphocytes which are able to destroy their targets by antibody-dependent cell-mediated cytotoxicity. Possess Fc receptors.

Langerhans cell: a type of dendritic cell found in the skin, bearing Fc receptors and MHC class II molecules, that is an antigen-presenting cell.

Large granular lymphocytes (LGLs): lymphoid cells that are defined by morphological criteria. They contain cytoplasmic lysosomes, and may act as natural killer (NK) or K cells.

Lymph node: one of many glands spread throughout the body, connected by lymph vessels, containing lymphocytes and APCs; these are the places where lymphocytes become activated against antigens and where memory cells reside.

Lymphokine-activated killer cells (LAK): killer and natural killer cells which, when activated by IL-2, exhibit more effective killing of their target cells.

Lymphocyte: a cell that has the capacity, because it has a unique surface receptor molecule, to react to antigen; these are the cells that make specific immune responses and are of three types, B cells, T cells and LGLs.

Lymphokines: a generic term for cytokines produced by activated lymphocytes, especially T cells, that act as intercellular mediators of the immune response.

Lysozyme: a crystalline, basic enzyme found in phagocytic cell granules, and in tears, saliva, and airway secretions, which digests mucopeptides of bacterial cell walls and therefore acts as a non-specific antibacterial agent.

Macrophage: a large cell derived from monocytes that can function as a phagocytic cell, antigen-presenting cell, and as a cytotoxic cell in ADCC.

Major histocompatibility complex (MHC): a set of genes found in all mammals (probably in all vertebrates) that regulate the activation of T cells and which through being markers of self, contribute to the tissue incompatibilities that cause graft rejection.

Mast cell: a bone marrow-derived cell found in tissues. It resembles peripheral blood basophils and bears Fc receptors for IgE. Very important in allergic (type I hypersensitivity) reactions.

Memory (immunologic): a characteristic of a specific immunological response in which secondary exposure to a given antigen produces a faster and greater response.

Monoclonal antibody: homogeneous antibody produced by a clone of B cells, often as a hybridoma.

Monocyte: a mononuclear, myeloid phagocytic cell whch circulates briefly in the bloodstream before migrating to the tissues to become a macrophage.

Mucous membranes (mucus): the lining cells of the respiratory, digestive and urogenital tracts that secrete the viscous fluid mucus; they are effectively on the outside of the body and are important in preventing microorganisms entering it.

Mutation: a change in the code of a gene; can occur either randomly or through exposure to radiation or certain chemicals (mutagens); may lead to a change in the structure of the protein coded by the mutated gene.

Natural killer (NK) cell: a large granular lymphocyte having cytotoxic ability. The cell lacks immunoglobulin or T-cell receptors but can recognize and destroy some tumour cells without MHC restriction.

Oncogenes: genes that control cell growth; if expressed inappropriately may cause cancer.

Opsonization: a process by which phagocytosis is facilitated by the deposition of opsonins (e.g. antibody and C3b) on the antigen.

Plasma cell: differentiated antibody-producing cell derived from an activated B cell.

Polymorphism: the expression of one of many (two or more) different alternative forms (alleles) of a particular gene at a particular locus (place) on the chromosome.

Polymorphonuclear neutrophil leucoyte (PMN): a circulating phagocytic granulocyte having cytotoxic ability; it has Fc receptors for immunoglobulin and can participate in ADCC.

Privileged sites: tissues where cells of the immune system normally do not go (e.g. cornea of the eye), in consequence graft rejection reactions against these tissues are usually very weak.

Prostaglandins: pharmacologically active derivatives of arachidonic acid. Different prostaglandins are capable of modulating cell mobility and immune responses.

Secondary response: the immune response which follows a second or subsequent encounter with a particular antigen.

Serum sickness: literally the immune response against repeated exposure to foreign serum proteins that leads to formation of immune complexes and damaging type III hypersensitivity reactions; can occur on repeated exposure to any foreign antigen.

Site-directed mutagenesis: a laboratory procedure that changes the sequence code of a particular part of a gene to create a protein with a new amino acid sequence that may cause structural and functional changes.

Specificity: the feature of the responses of lymphocytes characterized by their response only to the antigens with which their receptors interact; each lymphocyte has a receptor of subtly different structure and combining properties from all other lymphocytes.

Spleen: a secondary lymphoid organ connected with the blood supply that serves the same function as lymph nodes.

Stem cell: a continuously self-renewing cell that through division produces differentiated daughter cells with properties different from the original cell.

Superantigens: antigens which bind to the MHC outside of the peptide-binding groove and stimulate all or most of the T cells bearing particular T-cell receptor V regions.

T-cell receptor (TCR): the T cell antigen receptor consisting of either an α/β dimer (TCR2) or a γ/δ dimer (TCR1) associated with the CD3 molecular complex.

T cell: a lymphocyte that originated in the bone marrow and passed through the thymus during its development; reacts to antigen through possession of a specific receptor.

T-cytotoxic cell: a T cell capable of cytotoxicity against any target cell expressing the antigen to which it is specifically reactive.

T-helper cell: a $CD4^+$ T cell that produces interleukins to help B cells in making an antibody response; may also interact with $CD8^+$ T cells to aid their activation.

T-suppressor cell: a $CD8^+$ T cell that suppresses the immune function of other T cells or B cells.

Thrombocytopenia: a reduction in the number of platelets circulating in the blood.

Thymus: the gland situated in the thorax which is the site where T cells mature and achieve immune competence.

Tissue typing: laboratory procedures that allow the identification of antigens (especially HLA polymorphisms) on tissues and cells that may be important in transplant rejection and in genetic associations of diseases.

Transplantation antigen: any antigen on a tissue against which an immune response may be made when that tissue is transplanted to another individual; in humans the HLA and the ABO blood group system act in this way.

Vaccination: the intentional process of exposing an individual to an infectious organism (usually made innocuous in some way) with the intention of establishing a state of immunity to the organism.

INDEX